Contents

Executive Summary 6

Introduction 6

Potential "Digital" Healthcare Disparities 6

EHR Technical Considerations 7

Design and Development Guidelines 7

EHR Evaluation Guidelines 8

EHR Monitoring Guidelines 10

Research Guidelines 11

Conclusions 11

1   Introduction 13

2   Potential "Digital" Healthcare Disparities 15

2.1   History of Healthcare Disparities 15

2.2   Current Data 16

2.3   Causes and Determinants 16

2.4   National Trends 17

2.5   Provider Use of Electronic Tools in Healthcare Delivery 18

2.5.1   Provider Related Opportunities to Address Healthcare Disparities through Use of Electronic Tools 19

2.5.2   Patient and Caregiver Opportunities to Reduce Disparities through Use of Electronic Tools   20

2.6   EHR Related Human Factors Risk Characteristics among Target Populations at Highest Risk for Healthcare Disparities 20

2.6.1   Low Socioeconomic Status Groups 20

2.6.2   Non Native English Speakers or those with Limited English Proficiency 21

2.6.3   People Living with Disabilities 22

2.6.4   Seniors and the Elderly 26

2.6.5   Racial and Ethnic Minorities 28

3   EHR Technical Considerations of Healthcare Disparities 29

3.1.1   The EHR Development Life Cycle 29

3.1.2   The Potential of EHR Technical Design Issues to Impact Healthcare Disparities ... 34

4   Technical Guidance and Recommendations 35

4.1   EHR Design and Development Guidelines 35

4.1.1   Conduct Comprehensive Formative and Summative Testing with a Reasonable Set of Representative End Users 35

4.1.2 Report Results of the Tests in Common Industry Format (CIF) for EHR Usability Test Reports 36

4.1.3 Accommodate as Many EHR Users as Possible Using Universal Design Principles 36

4.1.4 Include Disparities Oriented Use Cases as Part of the EHR Design and Development Process 37

4.2 EHR Evaluation Guidelines 38

4.2.1 Require Documentation of Formative and Summative Testing with a Reasonable Set of Representative Target Users as a Prerequisite for EHR Evaluation 38

4.2.2 Require Documentation of Product Features Designed to Increase Usability and Accessibility or Documentation of a Lack of Need for any Accommodation among a Reasonable Set of Target Users 38

4.2.3 Require the Development of EHR Operation, Safety, Customer Support and Educational Materials that are Culturally and Linguistically Appropriate for a Reasonable Set of Representative Target Users as a Prerequisite for EHR Evaluation Process 38

4.2.4 Include User Requirements in Product Specifications as a Prerequisite for EHR Certification 41

4.3 EHR Evaluation and Monitoring Guidelines 41

4.3.1 Include Evaluation of EHR Impact on a Target Set of Healthcare Disparities Indicators as a Part of the EHR Effectiveness, Post Adoption and Health Impact Evaluation 41

4.3.2 Implement a National EHR Product Registry 42

4.4 EHR Research Guidelines 43

4.4.1 Support Human Factors Research Regarding the Potential Impact, Opportunities and Barriers for EHRs to Reduce Healthcare Disparities 43

4.4.2 Evaluate the Human Factors Implications of Integrating Patient-Oriented Functionality into EHRs 43

4.4.3 Support the Development of Evidence-Based Criteria for Voluntary Population-Oriented Product Certifications 43

4.4.4 Evaluate Potential Differences in Information Design Needs, the Impact of These Differences and Opportunities for Accommodation across User Populations 43

4.4.5 Evaluate the Human Factors Implications of Increased Stress (Workload Induced, User Environment Induced, Rural/Urban Residence etc) on EHR Accessibility, Usability, User Experience and Health Outcomes 44

4.4.6 Evaluate the Human Factors Implications of the Emerging EHR Health IT Workforce Working in Non Clinical Practice Settings (Home, Long Term Care Facility etc) on EHR Accessibility, Usability, User Experience and Health Outcomes. 44

5   Conclusions 44

Glossary 45

NISTIR 7769

Human Factors Guidance to Prevent Healthcare Disparities with the Adoption of EHRs

Michael C. Gibbons
Johns Hopkins University

Svetlana Z. Lowry
Information Access Division
Information Technology Laboratory
National Institute of Standards and Technology

Matthew T. Quinn
Information Access Division
Information Technology Laboratory
National Institute of Standards and Technology

February 2011

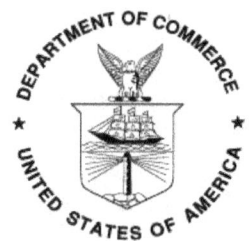

U.S. Department of Commerce
Gary Locke, Secretary

National Institute of Standards and Technology
Patrick D. Gallagher, Director

Healthcare Consumers 45

Patients 45

Providers 45

Culture.. 45

Culturally and Linguistically Appropriate Services (CLAS)............................ 45

Culturally and Linguistically Appropriate Services in Health Care 45

Healthcare Disparities.. 47

Safety Net Providers 47

Usability.. 48

User-Centered Design... 48

Universal Accessibility 49

Universal Usability 50

Human Factors Guidance to Prevent Healthcare Disparities with the Adoption of EHRs

Executive Summary

Introduction

This report is derived from several widely recognized international standards and the current scientific literature. It is intended for EHR system designers, developers, system architects and system engineers.

The advances in Information Technology (IT) that have been transforming our society have tremendous potential to improve healthcare in areas such as clinical care, administrative transactions, public health, professional education, biomedical research and consumer health (1). In fact, it has been suggested that information technology must play a central role in the redesign of the health care system, if substantial improvement in healthcare quality is to be achieved (1). There is also a growing interest in understanding the potential role of health IT in addressing healthcare disparities (2-4). In order to adequately and appropriately evaluate the potential of health IT to address healthcare disparities, health IT adoption and utilization barriers must be evaluated and understood. In addition, barriers must be considered from the perspective of all potential EHR users. These include the medical provider, support staff, patients, family members and caregivers. Finally, the impact of the environment in which the technology is used must be understood (e.g. hospital/clinic and home/community). Barriers, issues or problems in any one of these areas could impact health IT adoption, utilization and ultimately outcomes. If the nature of the problems are such that one population benefits more than another, national adoption of health IT could actually increase existing healthcare disparities or potentially even create new ones.

The purpose of this report is to provide technical guidance regarding the design and development of EHR systems, which will help to prevent the creation or exacerbation of healthcare disparities with the national adoption and utilization of EHR systems.

Potential "Digital" Healthcare Disparities

Several national healthcare reform efforts have called for an increasing role of health IT in healthcare delivery as a way to improve efficiency and quality while reducing healthcare costs. (1) To date, much of the attention regarding health IT in healthcare has been focused on the role of EHRs, Health Information Exchange (HIE), telemedicine, Computerized Physician Order Entry (CPOE) systems, e-prescribing and electronic radiologic systems. While national adoption data are limited for most forms of health IT, the most recent data for EHRs indicate that EHR adoption in U.S. medical offices is approximately 36.1% (5).

Within this context, the role of health IT in addressing healthcare disparities has only recently begun to receive consideration (2;4;6). There is great need for federal coordination and integration across multiple agencies particularly in the area of technical guidelines and standards that will help ensure broad EHR accessibility and usability and thereby reduce the possibility of creating or exacerbating healthcare disparities with the roll out, adoption and acceptance of EHRs and other emerging health IT products.

Several target populations are at increased risk for EHR related healthcare disparities. These include patients of low socioeconomic status and/or limited English proficiency. Patients living with disabilities, individuals over the age of 65, as well as racial and ethnic minorities are also at increased risk of experiencing EHR related healthcare disparities. They are more likely to lack access to a regular source of healthcare. Significant mistrust of the medical system has also been documented among these populations. This mistrust contributes to an increased likelihood of patient refusal and poor adherence to provider recommendations. It also contributes to poor doctor-patient communication which leads to limited patient comprehension or confusion regarding healthcare information.

Without EHR design accommodations, these patient contingents will likely also be associated with several types of human factors risks that may limit comprehension and understanding of EHR information and reduce EHR accessibility or usability. These problems will inevitably lead to poor EHR user experiences and limited EHR adoption among high risk patients. They may also contribute to poor user experiences among safety net providers (See Glossary) who practice in under-resourced settings or otherwise care for large numbers of these underserved patients.

Before applying an IT solution, it is important to know what disparities related factors are amenable to IT solutions.

EHR Technical Considerations

There are stages in the EHR design process, where human factors considerations could impact EHR usability among users at high risk for experiencing healthcare disparities. Current evidence of vendor practices suggest Human Factors Engineering (HFE) and ergonomics design principles are not systematically and formally employed during the EHR design process (7).

Robust user-centered design process, based on comprehensive user-centered task analysis and the explicit characterization of unique user experience requirements, living environment (use context) requirements, cultural requirements and EHR interface requirements is needed. This will help ensure the development of accessible and usable EHR systems for target end users at increased risk of experiencing healthcare disparities and safety net providers caring for these patients.

Design and Development Guidelines

Universal usability approach will significantly reduce the likelihood of healthcare disparities with the adoption of EHRs. Generally, these recommendations focus on equipping the EHR design team with the information necessary to understand potential healthcare disparities challenges related to use of the EHR. These recommendations also focus on ensuring that this information is then used to improve EHR system usability via the iterative design process.

Conduct comprehensive formative and summative testing with a reasonable set of representative target users
To help ensure broad EHR accessibility and usability, it is imperative that usability testing involve those who are likely to be using the system.

Designers and Developers should use the Common Industry Format (CIF) for EHR usability test reports
The Common Industry Format (CIF) for Usability Test Reports is intended for use in reporting the results of summative usability testing (8). Usability of EHR systems is a key factor in predicting successful deployment. EHR system developers and manufacturers must subject EHRs to usability testing at various stages in a product's development. Testing should involve

(1) subjects who are representative of the target population of EHR users, (2) representative tasks, and (3) measures of efficiency, effectiveness and subjective satisfaction.

Accommodate as many EHR users as possible via the use of universal design principles
To ensure that as many potential EHR users as possible are able to use emerging EHR systems safely and effectively, a Universal Design strategy (See Glossary) should be adopted. Accommodating a broader spectrum of users and user contexts will require designers to consider a wider range of designs. Many of the design accommodations can be incorporated without significant impact on developmental time or expense. Once completed, these improvements often lead to innovations that benefit all users (9).

Include disparities-oriented use case scenarios and user contexts as part of the EHR design and developmental planning process
In an effort to reduce the likelihood of design flaws that disproportionately impact health patients from healthcare disparities populations or safety net providers it will be important to enhance development process by considering disparities-oriented use case scenarios and user contexts to guide the planning effort. In the absence of demonstrated disparities expertise on the part of EHR designers and developers, it cannot be assumed that all the necessary considerations can or will be made. Disparities-oriented use cases may include:

1) Adult caregiver of a senior relative use case

In many families, adult children caring for elderly parents is becoming increasingly common. This may be even more likely among patients from disparity populations who may lack resources to provide alternate care arrangements for their aging relative. The cognitive and physical demands and stress of care giving combined with childrearing, homemaking and also additional employment may create critical challenges for the safe and effective use of EHRs. In other words, the consideration of these broader patient user contexts, may be as critical for understanding EHR usability by patients, as understanding clinical workflows in the hospital is for understanding provider EHR usability.

2) Patient/Caregiver with limited English proficiency use case

Providing care to patients with limited English proficiency creates challenges for all involved parties. This is no less true in the context of EHR-mediated care. Misunderstandings or confusion caused by a poorly designed EHR, in the context of marginal English proficiency, may prove more challenging and more difficult to even detect than complete inability to use the available system unless these types of use cases are employed.

3) EHR use in the context of doctor-patient cross cultural or communications barriers use case

In some cultures, major decision making is considered a family or at least a combined activity between a husband and a wife. However, informed consent and access to EHR information is currently considered largely from the Western perspective (i.e. single users and individual rights). Usability, user experience and satisfaction implications with the use of such an EHR are not likely to be optimal. There should be design accommodations that could help address the challenges created by these cultural differences.

EHR Evaluation Guidelines
Documentation of summative testing with a reasonable set of representative target users should be required

To ensure that all end user contingents are defined and user requirements are implemented in the product development cycle, summative testing report in CIF format should be available.

Require documentation of product features designed to ensure accessibility; and any accommodations needed for users with disabilities

To ensure that vendors are making appropriate design enhancements specifically for the purpose of improving identified limitations among target users, it is recommended that documentation of included product features be provided as part of EHR evaluation process.

Require the development of EHR operation, safety, customer support and educational materials that are culturally and linguistically appropriate for a reasonable set of representative target users

Writing clear EHR functionality related system messages and instructional materials is critically important as an increasing variety of users adopts EHRs. The following specific recommendations are made for instructional materials for both paper and electronic formats (10). These should not be viewed as an exhaustive nor comprehensive set of recommendations. Rather these can be considered as a starting point for the development of more effective and usable EHR instructional materials.

1) Put instructions where (at specific point on the screen) they are needed – not all together at the top of the page.

2) Put instructions above/before they are needed – not after.

3) Put instructions in logical order first task, first; last task, last.

4) Put warnings about consequences before – not after – the user is likely to act.

5) Do not highlight the action option until EHR users have been given all available options.

6) The order of buttons must match the order of the instructions.

7) Start each instruction on a new line.

8) Write directly to the EHR user.

9) Keep each instruction as short as possible.

10) Watch the tone. Help EHR users, don't threaten them.

11) Write in the positive.

12) Put the context before the action.

13) Be consistent in the language of the instructions.

14) Do not use gender-based pronouns.

15) Use simple English words.

16) Be consistent in the language that is used.

17) Do not use technical, computer jargon.

18) Be explicit in naming buttons.

19) Cover all important situations.

20) Consider EHR users' likely mistakes.

21) Understand the audience for messages about EHR problems.

22) Understand the context for messages about problems.

23) Messages and instructional material should be designed and tested for specific clinician or patient, caregiver and consumer use cases and contexts.

Include user requirements in product specifications

To help ensure that the best match is achieved between EHR features and user needs, it is recommended that user requirements be included in all EHR product specifications. This will allow potential users to make informed choices regarding the applicability of a given EHR product for a given set of user needs. Common Industry Specification for Usability–Requirements (CISU-R) http://zing.ncsl.nist.gov/iusr/documents/whatistheCISUR.html

EHR Monitoring Guidelines

Include evaluation of EHR impact on a target set of healthcare disparities indicators as a part of the EHR effectiveness, post adoption and health impact evaluation

All efforts to document the effectiveness of EHR systems should also include specific investigation of the EHR impact on healthcare disparities. The EHR healthcare disparities indicator set has to be defined. Once defined, it should be used as the basis for conducting ongoing healthcare disparities impact assessments. This work should be supplemented by additional qualitative research among safety net providers and patients from disparities populations, to provide additional information regarding the nature, character, quality, magnitude and emergence of new determinants or elimination of current determinants of Healthcare disparities impacted by EHR adoption and use.

Implement a National EHR Product Registry

Given the number and diversity of EHR developers and vendors as well as the diverse and dynamic needs of potential EHR users, it is recommended that a National EHR Product Registry be developed for all certified EHR products and other products which in the future are integrated into or otherwise linked with an EHR system. This registry should have standardized reporting requirements as outlined below. This registry would provide significant scientific research, consumer research, product safety and patient educational benefit, for potential EHR customers, users and providers.

EHR Product reporting recommendations targeting EHR Vendors

Standardize EHR technical elements & design feature reporting

Certified EHR vendors should be required to report a standard set of technical and design features. The reporting requirements should be developed through a consensus driven process of public and private partners including Healthcare disparities, disabilities, and underserved population's expertise. Reported data should be publicly available.

EHR product evaluation reporting

Certified EHR vendors should be required to report a standard set of EHR evaluation information. In the future this should include any target user-oriented voluntary certifications received by the EHR product. Evaluation information should include information about user requirements and product specifications.

EHR Product reporting recommendations targeting Providers and Healthcare Systems

Adverse event reporting

The National EHR Product Registry should facilitate voluntary, provider and healthcare system adverse event reporting.

Provider Feedback

The registry should also facilitate provider feedback regarding the EHR challenges problems, malfunctions, errors experienced while using the system.

EHR Product reporting recommendations targeting Patient, Consumers and Caregivers
Patient education
The National EHR Product Registry should provide culturally and linguistically appropriate patient educational information regarding certified EHR and associated technology. The information should be supplied by the product vendors but should comply with recognized federal standards for providing Culturally Linguistically Appropriate Services (See Glossary) and communicating information to diverse populations (11).

Consumer feedback
The National EHR Product Registry should facilitate patient and consumer feedback about EHR systems.

Research Guidelines

Evaluate potential differences in information design needs, the impact of these differences and opportunities for accommodation across user populations
It is not clear whether or not different populations of users based on race/ethnicity, culture or socioeconomic status have differing information design needs and whether or not such needs can impact healthcare disparities. Because information architecture is at the heart of any EHR design, usability and understanding, research in this area may have significant import for addressing healthcare disparities via EHR systems.

Evaluate the Human Factors implications of increased stress (workload induced, user environment induced, rural/urban residence, etc) on EHR accessibility, usability, user experience and health outcomes
To date, most of the research regarding stress and human-computer interaction has been done in the context of the work environment. However, as healthcare is increasingly being delivered in the home and in community-based settings and as patients increasingly become engaged in their EHRs, more research needs to be done to understand the potential impact of the home environment on EHR accessibility, usability, user experience and health outcomes.

Evaluate the Human Factors implications of the emerging EHR Health IT workforce working in non-clinical practice settings (home, long-term care facility, etc) on EHR accessibility, usability, user experience and health outcomes.
A myriad of support personnel will inevitably be EHR system users. These include clinical office/practice managers, receptionist/schedulers and technical support personnel. Without these individuals involved, many providers would not be able to accomplish needed EHR data entry or report/summary requirements. Also there is an emerging health workforce comprised of those individuals who provide or support care primarily in home and community settings (Community Health Workers, Patient Navigators etc). It is likely that in order to maintain appropriate oversight and management, as well as quality assurance and efficiency, these individuals will increasingly be using wireless handheld and tablet or laptop-based mobile devices to input data into the EHR in real time, in the field, at the "point of care". The implications of this emerging workforce on health, healthcare outcomes and healthcare disparities need to be evaluated.

Conclusions

Significant scientific evidence attests to the fact that healthcare disparities exist, they are intractable and associated with increased healthcare costs, premature morbidity and excess mortality. Wide adoption and meaningful use of EHR systems by providers and patients may impact healthcare disparities. Predicting exact impacts is a challenge because the effects of EHR utilization on Healthcare disparities are likely to multiple, nuanced, cumulative and at times indirect. Disparities could improve, if EHR use and benefits are equitably distributed across user populations. On the other hand, disparities could worsen, if some providers are not able to use EHRs or some patients are not able to benefit from them.

The field of human factors engineering and ergonomics has made considerable contributions to our understanding of the possible barriers and potential solutions needed to ensure broad accessibility and usability of emerging EHR systems. Unfortunately, most of this knowledge and expertise does not appear to be routinely considered during the EHR design and development process (7). In addition, little research along these lines can be found in the disparities literature. Few studies of EHR usability or health impact have been done from a healthcare disparities perspective. As such, much more research is warranted. There is also considerable need for federal policy leadership in this area. This leadership will help ensure that all providers are able to use EHRs and also help ensure that all patients are able to benefit from EHR use. Finally, given what is already known, much can be done now to reduce the risk of creating or exacerbating healthcare disparities. Product enhancements can be made by addressing key disparities-related design issues and by incorporating human factors engineering principles into the EHR design and development process. Significant progress along these lines, will inevitably improve provider EHR adoption, help lead to reductions in healthcare disparities among affected populations and catalyze improvements in healthcare quality for all.

1 Introduction

The Health Information Technology for Economic and Clinical Health Act's (HITECH Act's) provisions to drive adoption and meaningful use of Electronic Health Records (EHRs) holds great promise in supporting improvements in the quality, efficiency and effectiveness of care delivery. Replacing paper-based processes with electronic ones will have profound implications on both how care is delivered and how workers in healthcare organizations perform their jobs.

Recently, several national healthcare improvement efforts (12;13) have fostered interest in the use of health IT in healthcare. These consider information technology as playing a central role in the redesign of the healthcare system if a substantial improvement in healthcare quality is to be achieved (1). Within this context, the role of health IT in addressing healthcare disparities has only recently begun to receive consideration (2;4;6). In order to adequately and appropriately evaluate the potential of health IT to address healthcare disparities, health IT adoption and utilization barriers must be understood. It will also be important to understand the potential opportunities to effectively address healthcare disparities through health IT. Such analyses will enable an evidence-based approach to the design, development and deployment of appropriate electronic tools and provide the best foundation for using health IT to help address healthcare disparities.

With the introduction of EHRs, it is vitally important that EHR developers and healthcare organizations design, develop and implement EHRs in such a way that supports meaningful use by all users, including those with disabilities, and not introduce a "digital divide."

While EHRs are principally used by healthcare workers, patients interact with these systems directly (e.g. shared use of a display in an exam room) and indirectly through their outputs (e.g. copies of patient records, discharge instructions). To gain the intended benefits of this technology, EHR systems must display or deliver information in a manner and structure that is suitable for their needs and preferences. Therefore, it is vitally important that EHR developers and healthcare organizations implement meaningful use requirements and other functionalities involving patients in a way that supports the patients, populations and communities that they serve.

This paper will provide technical guidance for EHR developers and healthcare organizations regarding the design, development and implementation of EHR systems to prevent the creation or exacerbation of "digital disparities" with the national adoption and utilization of EHR systems, in the workplace and among patients. Through identification and application of best practices, guidance and standards in software usability and accessibility, system developers and healthcare organizations can ensure that EHR system support meaningful use by users that reflect the make-up of the healthcare workforce and patient-base.

Significant, pervasive and intractable healthcare disparities have been convincingly documented at all levels of the healthcare system. A large body of work has demonstrated the existence of these disparities across racial and ethnic lines (14). However they can also be demonstrated across individuals living with disabilities, people of low socioeconomic status and among those with limited English proficiency. In addition, several national trends suggest the scope and magnitude of these disparities are likely to increase. Healthcare disparities are associated with poorer health outcomes, premature death and increased personal and healthcare system costs (15;16).

There is evidence that EHR systems represent one promising way of enhancing the quality of healthcare, reducing waste, fraud and inefficiency in the healthcare system, improving health outcomes and reducing healthcare disparities. Less evident, however, is the ability of all healthcare organizations to use health IT effectively in the achievement of these goals, given their specific contexts and populations served. Most of the focus within the healthcare system has been on the potential of EHR systems and other decision support tools for healthcare providers. Interestingly though, outside the healthcare system, much of the focus has been on patient- and consumer-oriented (See Glossary) decision support tools. Indeed, it is envisioned, that future EHR systems will provide decision support to healthcare providers and patients, alike.

EHRs should be designed to take account of the people who will use them. Therefore, all relevant user groups should be identified. It is likely to be a potential contributor to the development of healthcare disparities. The extent to which products are usable and accessible depends on the context of use. The context of use is a major source of information for establishing requirements and an essential input to the design process (17).

2 Potential "Digital" Healthcare Disparities

2.1 History of Healthcare Disparities

Over the last two decades, scientific research examining variability in clinical practice patterns, has begun to accumulate (18;19). In the mid eighties, the report of the Secretary's Task Force on Black and Minority Health (20) highlighted, for the first time, at a national level in the United States, the fact that the health of African-Americans and minorities significantly lagged behind that of Whites. Upon closer examination it was revealed that problems associated with quality healthcare and racial and ethnic healthcare differences were in fact linked. Additionally, it became recognized that certain community, environment and societal factors including stress (21;22), early life experiences (23), social capital (24), and income inequality (25;26) seemed to exert significant effects on health, independent of personal behavior (27). Several efforts were undertaken to clarify the impact of these "nonmedical" factors on healthcare outcomes. By the late 1990's, the scientific evidence seemed to indicate that issues of healthcare disparities, clinical practice variation, substandard medical care and socio-environmental determinants of health, were all associated with the quality of healthcare experienced by patients (3). This work culminated with the 2003 release of a report entitled "Unequal Treatment: Confronting Racial and Ethnic Disparities in Healthcare" (1). This report found that within the United States, even among individuals with access to care, significant racial and ethnic disparities existed. The report also found that these disparities were associated with higher morbidity and mortality and were therefore unjustifiable (14). This report has subsequently spurred significant local and national effort to address these disparities. While some progress has been made, much more work is needed to enable significant, sustained improvements.

Generally, the causes of healthcare disparities are held to be related to three sets of factors. Firstly, patient related factors that include lack of a regular source of care, poor patient-provider communications, mistrust in the medical system, cultural insensitivity and inability to understand medical providers. Secondly, provider related factors that include bias and clinical uncertainty when interacting with racial and ethnic minority patients. Language barriers between providers and patients also may play a role in the establishment of healthcare disparities. Finally, healthcare system factors include the fragmentary nature of healthcare delivery and the organization of the healthcare establishment as well as financial incentives. Despite significant effort, healthcare disparities are not improving. In addition, without effective intervention, over the course of the next few years, healthcare disparities are expected to increase. This increase will further strain on the fragile and challenged US Healthcare system.

The development of computer technology has created an information gap that has grown faster and wider over recent years. As healthcare systems and providers rely more on information from the Internet to guide day-to-day care, the disparity between the information "haves and have nots" expands. Awareness of the disparity and its impact on healthcare is the first step in narrowing the information gap. Reasons for the gap are complex and multi-factorial, as are the solutions. The information gap will likely remain wherever there is poverty, illiteracy, or indifference. In terms of healthcare, this can mean disparity in information available to healthcare providers and the continuation of outdated, less effective treatment approaches. According to Fowler (2003), "The feedback loop between research and practice will become smaller, tighter, and faster" (p. 11), resulting in healthcare providers having greater and quicker access to the latest healthcare information. For the disconnected public, it can mean less awareness of health problems and how to manage them, and less self-empowerment. (28)

2.2 Current Data

Today, evaluating and addressing healthcare disparities is considered an integral part of improving healthcare quality and outcomes. The National Healthcare Disparities Report (NHDR) is an annual report commissioned by congress to monitor the nation's progress toward eliminating healthcare disparities among various racial, ethnic and income groups and other priority populations (29). Three key themes emerged in the 2009 NHDR. Firstly, disparities related to race, ethnicity, and socioeconomic status still pervade the American healthcare system. Although varying in magnitude by condition and population, disparities are observed in almost all aspects of healthcare, including: 1) across all dimensions of healthcare quality (including effectiveness, patient safety, timeliness, and patient-centeredness); 2) across all dimensions of access to care (including facilitators and barriers to care and healthcare utilization); 3) across many levels and types of care (including preventive care, treatment of acute conditions, and management of chronic diseases); 4) across many clinical conditions (cancer, diabetes, end stage renal disease, heart disease, HIV disease, mental health and substance abuse, and respiratory diseases); 5) across many care settings (including primary care, home healthcare, hospice care, emergency departments, hospitals, and nursing homes); 6) within many subpopulations (including women, children, older adults, residents of rural areas, and individuals with disabilities and other special healthcare needs) (29).

Secondly the report indicated that previously identified disparities are not improving. Measures of quality include effectiveness (the percentage of patients with a disease or condition who get recommended care), patient safety, and timeliness. Measures of access to care include health insurance coverage, utilization of general health services, and barriers to care (29).

Finally the report suggests that some disparities merit particular attention, especially care for cancer, heart failure, and pneumonia. Findings from the 2009 NHDR show that disparities in care for cancer, heart failure, and pneumonia exist across populations. Although quality of hospital care for heart failure and pneumonia has improved overall, care for Whites continues to improve at a higher rate than for minority populations. Thus, quality improvement has not necessarily translated to disparities reduction, which is critical for high-quality care. Low rates of colorectal cancer screening and other cancer screenings among minorities may be due to cultural attitudes and patient perceptions, such as, the belief that screening is not necessary. In addition, patients may have problems paying for follow-up visits to complete screening and may have logistical problems getting to appointments. Similarly, pneumococcal vaccination rates may be lower for Blacks and Asians because of distrust in the effectiveness of vaccines and perceptions that vaccines are not necessary (29).

2.3 Causes and Determinants

Before applying an IT solution, it is important to know what disparities related factors are amenable to IT solutions. As such, it is necessary to first present a short discussion of the major determinants of healthcare disparities.

Determinants of healthcare disparities exist on at least three levels. These include patient-level, provider-level and healthcare system factors. In terms of patient-level factors, racial and ethnic minority patients are more likely to refuse recommended services, adhere poorly to treatment, and delay seeking care. These behaviors and attitudes can develop as a result of a poor cultural match between minority patients and their providers, mistrust, misunderstanding of provider instructions, poor prior interactions with healthcare systems, or simply from a lack of knowledge of how to best use healthcare services (14). However these differences in refusal rates are small and cannot fully account for observed disparities. The responses of racial and ethnic minority patients to healthcare providers are also a potential source of disparities. If patients convey mistrust, refuse treatment, or comply poorly with treatment, providers may become less engaged in the treatment process. Patients then, are less likely to receive more vigorous treatments and services. Patients' and providers' behavior and attitudes may therefore influence each other, but reflect the attitudes, expectations, and perceptions that each has developed in a context where race and ethnicity are often more salient than these participants may realize (14).

Provider-related factors include provider bias (or prejudice), clinical uncertainty when interacting with minority patients, and provider beliefs (or stereotypes) about a given patient may influence healthcare disparities (14). The doctor can be viewed as operating with prior beliefs that will be different according to age, gender, socioeconomic status, and race or ethnicity of the patient. When these beliefs are considered alongside the information gained in a clinical encounter, both may influence medical decisions (14). If the physician has difficulty accurately understanding the symptoms or other diagnostic information, then he or she is likely to place greater weight on his or her beliefs, biases and stereotypes. The consequence is that treatment decisions and patients' needs are potentially less well matched and may tend to increase healthcare disparities (14).

Finally, healthcare system factors including language barriers pose a problem for many patients. Nearly 14 million Americans are not proficient in English. As many as one in five patients speak Spanish. Similarly, time pressures on physicians may hamper their ability to accurately assess the symptoms of minority patients, especially when cultural or linguistic barriers are present. Perhaps more significantly, changes in the financing and delivery of healthcare services including cost-control efforts and the movement to managed care, may pose greater barriers to care for racial and ethnic minorities than for non-minorities. This may happen through incentives to increase efficiency or reduce expenditures/costs (14).

2.4 National Trends

Several population trends form the basis for growing concern that healthcare disparities will increase in coming years, producing significant stress on an already challenged healthcare system. First, the U.S. population is expected to reach approximately 400 million. The Census Bureau projects that the U.S. population will continue to grow, to 420 million persons by year 2050. This growth is due to increasing survival rates, declining mortality rates, high fertility rates and significant immigration (30).

Second, the proportion of seniors in the U.S. population (aged ≥ 65) is expected to increase from just over 12% in 2000 to approximately 20% in 2030. This translates into an increase from 35 million to approximately 71 million seniors (31). The number of persons aged >80 years is expected to increase from about 9 million in 2000 to 19 million in 2030. These changes are also occurring because of an increase in the average life span combined with elevated fertility rates after World War II (the "Baby Boom") (31).

Third, the United States, like other developed countries, has experienced a shift in the leading causes of death, from infectious diseases and acute illnesses to chronic diseases and degenerative illnesses. In 2001, the leading causes of death in the United States were primarily cardiovascular diseases and cancer. The leading causes of death around the time of the birth of the United States were primarily infectious and parasitic diseases (31). In the United States, approximately 80% of all seniors have at least one chronic condition, and 50% have at least two (31).

Fourth, the United States is also becoming more racially and ethnically diverse. This is occurring primarily due to immigration. Although most immigrants tend to be young adults, U.S. immigration policy has favored the entry of parents and other family members of these young immigrants. At the same time, major racial and ethnic groups age at different rates due to fertility, mortality, and immigration differences within these groups (30).

While about 81% of the population was White in 2000, that figure is projected to fall to 72% by year 2050. Increases will be most dramatic for Asians and for persons in the "other races" category (which includes American Indians and Alaska Natives, Native Hawaiians and other Pacific Islanders, and individuals who identify with two or more races). Between 2000 and 2050, the number of Asians is expected to increase by 22.7 million, an increase of 213%, while the number in the "all other races" (which includes persons who identify with two or more races) category will increase by 15.3 million, or 217%. The population of Hispanic or Latino origin is projected to steadily increase as a percentage of the total U.S. population through 2050, rising from 12.6% in 2000 to 24.4% in 2050 (30).

Taken together, these trends (the increasing population size, increasing proportions of racial and ethnic minorities, the increased prevalence of chronic diseases and significantly increasing numbers of older persons) represent a challenge for the U.S. healthcare system. As the U.S. population ages and becomes more diverse, the social, medical and economic demands on the health and social care systems will grow. Increasing demand will tend to also further increase healthcare costs. As such, critical questions remain regarding the best mechanisms for health system organization, delivery, access and healthcare financing. Those patients and populations with fewer resources to deal with these challenges (seniors, immigrant, minorities, the poor and disabled) will be disproportionately affected, thereby increasing the gaps in healthcare access, quality and outcomes between the underserved and the general population. (30).

2.5   Provider Use of Electronic Tools in Healthcare Delivery

To date, much of the attention regarding health IT in healthcare has been focused on the role of EHRs, HIE, telemedicine, CPOE systems, e-prescribing and electronic radiologic systems. While national adoption data are limited for most forms of health IT, the most recent data for EHRs indicate that EHR adoption in U.S. medical offices is 36.1% (18). Providers primarily use EHR systems for electronic notes, viewing/ordering labs/x-rays and e-prescribing. Several factors tend to be associated with higher EHR adoption rates. These include group practices with a larger number of physicians, a higher number of available exam rooms and higher daily patient volumes (5).

Data from the 2005 and 2006 National Ambulatory Medical Care Survey (NAMCS) and National Hospital Ambulatory Medical Care Survey (NHAMCS) indicate that EHR adoption is lower among providers serving Hispanic or Latino patients who are uninsured or rely on Medicaid. It also found lower EHR adoption among providers of uninsured non-Hispanic Black patients than for providers of privately insured non-Hispanic White patients. Primary care providers in private solo or small group practice have the lowest adoption rate (5.7 percent), whereas those in other office settings (including HMOs, faculty practice plans, and urgent care centers) have the highest adoption rate (38.3 percent) (32). A study has also shown that specialty physicians are more favorable towards adopting EHR systems than primary care physicians. The lower adoption rate among primary care physicians can be attributed to the complex workflows that exist in their offices leading to non-standardized workflow structures and practices.(33)

2.5.1 Provider Related Opportunities to Address Healthcare Disparities through Use of Electronic Tools

Several provider-level determinants of healthcare disparities may be impacted by health IT. For example, a major goal of many of the provider-oriented health IT tools is to make pertinent patient information available to providers at the point of care. This information help reduce clinical uncertainty related to certain unclear/incorrect patient information found in handwritten medical records. In the absence of needed information or in the presence of unclear/ambiguous data, providers may undervalue or under appreciate patient-specific information, over-weigh beliefs, assumptions, biases or stereotypes about certain types of patients (4). If the needed information is clearly presented to the clinician in the EHR, it should increase the use of clear and accurate patient information by obviating the need for relying on less appropriate data. Over time, this is likely to have the cumulative effect of promoting high quality personalized care across patients and reducing related healthcare disparities (4).

EHRs also provide physicians with information about appropriate treatment options, thus providing clinical decision support (4). Health IT tools, through reminders, quality reports or clinical benchmarking may also provide clinical decision support by generating feedback to providers regarding their clinical performance. Reminders and quality reports provide feedback to providers about the quality of care they provide to a particular patient during a clinical encounter or about the care they have provided to a group of patients over a time. If these reports include specific disparity indicators, it can help reduce those disparities by exposing unrecognized clinical practices which fall short of accepted standards and guidelines. These reports may also help by highlighting a provider's performance across all patients. Providers may then work to reduce identified disparities by focusing on those areas which need improvement (4).

Health IT tools like EHR systems, e-mail, e-consultation, e-prescribing and CPOE systems function to connect physicians with other healthcare professionals and other people (7). . They also facilitate reduction in healthcare disparities in patient care by providing ready access to the needed clinical knowledge for better diagnostic and therapeutic decisions. Other forms of health IT tools, including telemedicine, remote monitors and sensors, patient e-mail the internet and social media, connect providers and healthcare systems to their patients and caregivers (34). These tools may reduce disparities by providing education and support to disparity populations and by enabling access to care, otherwise unavailable. However, disparities tend to actually increase if these tools are used unevenly across populations, or they are designed in a way that precludes safe and appropriate use by patients and caregivers with limited English proficiency, limited educational backgrounds, disabilities or limited ability to access these tools (4).

Another way in which health IT tools that connect providers with patients may impact healthcare disparities is by enabling increased monitoring of essential and critical patient clinical parameters among racial and ethnic minority patients. Since many patients often fail to adequately monitor or self-mange their conditions, remote monitoring via patient sensor ("smart") technology, can enable direct delivery of patient data (e.g., glucose levels, weight, vital signs, falls, psychological or musculoskeletal stress/injury, etc.) to a device or even an EHR. These data (e.g.. blood sugar, weight gain/loss) could facilitate better clinical management and disease control resulting in lower complication rates (e.g., blindness, renal failure, limb loss) and delay in disease progression (e.g., diabetes, congestive heart failure) by potentially narrowing the disparities. These tools can also facilitate a more stable relationship between a patient and the provider by enabling patients to overcome barriers to regular communication and access to care or otherwise, in maintaining a patient-provider relationship. Having a regular source of care has been described as a significant determinant of healthcare disparities (35;36). By improving and stabilizing patient-provider communication and relationship, these tools may also help promote enhanced patient involvement in care, facilitate shared decision-making and strengthen patient-centered care. These factors are recognized as some other important determinants of healthcare disparities and also, essential for high quality healthcare (37-43).

2.5.2 Patient and Caregiver Opportunities to Reduce Disparities through Use of Electronic Tools

There are many new opportunities for patients and caregivers to utilize technology to manage their health and the care provided. The Institute of Medicine, Centers for Medicare and Medicaid Services and other bodies are beginning to emphasize that care should be provided not only during face-to-face visits, but also via a variety of formats. E-Health and health IT tools should be used to increase patient access, enhance patient engagement, re-engineer patient-centered care and foster the continuous healing relationships needed to appropriately manage chronic illnesses (1;44;45). These opportunities can potentially reduce the incidence or impact of healthcare disparities among affected populations by improving access to care.

Health IT tools designed primarily for patients could in the future, become important options to support patient health education. Due to the prevalence of health literacy challenges which occur disproportionately among minority populations, many patients appear to lack the necessary skills to fully understand or comprehend provider instructions, medication and healthcare product labels or adhere to complex self-management (46;47). Incomplete or partial understanding of health and healthcare issues may fuel lack of trust in the healthcare system. Mistrust has been linked to devaluing or disregarding provider instructions and patient non-adherence among certain disparity populations (35;48-52). As such, technology based approaches to providing culturally, linguistically and cognitively appropriate and accessible health education may represent one way to build patient trust, increase access to needed health care services, enhance patient engagement in their healthcare management and decision-making and ultimately improve disparate outcomes (3).

To date, much of the patient-oriented focus on health IT has been on the role of Personal Health Record (PHR) systems. PHRs, majority of them being Internet-based, are tools that may be linked with the EHRs. They allow people to access, input, change, coordinate and control their health information. The major difference between a PHR and an EHR is the lack of patient access and control of the EHR (44). In addition, other patient-oriented health IT tools as well, promise to support patient's health-related behaviors. By enhancing social support and interaction, these tools may enhance medication adherence (reminders systems), patient-provider communication (EHR, emails), physician cultural competency (crowdsourcing technologies) and healthy lifestyles (location based social media). These, thereby reduce disparities particularly among racial and ethnic minority populations where utilization of social media and mobile applications is significantly higher than among the White populations (53;54).

2.6 EHR Related Human Factors Risk Characteristics among Target Populations at Highest Risk for Healthcare Disparities

2.6.1 Low Socioeconomic Status Groups

The U.S. Census Bureau reports that real median household income in the United States in 2009 was $49,777 which was unchanged from 2008. The nation's official poverty rate in 2009 was 14.3 percent, up from 13.2 percent in 2008. There were 43.6 million people living in poverty in 2009, up from 39.8 million in 2008 — the third consecutive annual increase. Households in the West and Northeast had the highest median household incomes. Also in 2009, the earnings of women who worked full time, year-round remained at 77% of that for corresponding men. On the other hand the real median earning of men who worked full time, year-round rose by 2.0

percent between 2008 and 2009, from $46,191 to $47,127. For women, the corresponding increase was slightly less at1.9 %, from $35,609 to $36,278 (55).

The poverty rate in 2009 was the highest since 1994, but was 8.1 percentage points lower than the poverty rate in 1959, the first year for which poverty estimates are available. The number of people in poverty in 2009 is the largest number in the 51 years for which poverty estimates are available. In 2009, the family poverty rate and the number of families in poverty were 11.1 percent and 8.8 million, respectively, up from 10.3 percent and 8.1 million in 2008. Finally, the poverty rate and the number in poverty increased across all types of families: married-couple families (5.8 percent and 3.4 million in 2009 from 5.5 percent and 3.3 million in 2008); female-householder-with-no-husband-present families (29.9 percent and 4.4 million in 2009 from 28.7 percent and 4.2 million in 2008) and for male-householder-no-wife-present families (16.9 percent and 942,000 in 2009 from 13.8 percent and 723,000 in 2008) (55).

Individuals from low socioeconomic status groups are at increased risk of healthcare disparities because they are much more likely than the general population to lack appropriate ongoing access to healthcare services. It is important to note that the risks extend to both providers and patients from low socioeconomic groups. Although individuals who come from low socioeconomic groups who then become healthcare providers often achieve a level of personal income above that which could be achieved otherwise, they also are more likely to practice in low socioeconomic status communities providing care in low resource facilities, providing care for the poor and uninsured. As such these providers are less likely to own, purchase or utilize EHRs (32). Thus the patients seen by these providers will be unable to access the benefits derived from receiving care from a provider who utilizes an EHR. In addition the low socioeconomic status patients and consumers themselves are much less likely to use or access information via an EHR or Personal Health Record (PHR) even if one is available (32;44;56).

2.6.2 Non Native English Speakers or those with Limited English Proficiency

Health literacy is defined as the ability to read and comprehend health-related materials (57). While health literacy depends in part on individuals' skills, it also depends on the complexity of health information and the way it is communicated (58). Only 12 percent of U.S. adults have high health literacy. Over a third of U.S. adults or approximately 77 million people would have difficulty with common health tasks, such as following directions on a prescription drug label or adhering to a childhood immunization schedule using a standard chart (58). Limited English proficiency rates are also prevalent among the poor, urban and minority populations (59). Studies of Limited English proficiency patients suggest that they are less likely to understand hospital discharge instructions or know essential information about diseases (60).

Conceptually, health literacy affects patients' ability to manage their health and influences their healthcare seeking behaviors. Patients with Limited English proficiency may find it difficult to understand, implement and adhere to their providers' recommendations. This is particularly important for patients with chronic conditions. Limited English proficiency may also limit a patient's ability to utilize emerging health technologies. Moreover, complex health information can overwhelm even individuals with proficient health literacy skills. Research has shown that health information often exceeds individuals' health literacy capabilities (58). Recent years have seen an increase in awareness of the mismatch between patients' skills and the health literacy demands that are placed on them. There is growing recognition that healthcare systems and professionals have a responsibility to accommodate and help improve patients' understanding (58).

Patients and caregivers with limited English proficiency are likely at increased risk of experiencing EHR usability or information comprehension problems, increased risk for inappropriate EHR utilization and less likely to achieve long term adoption of EHR systems.

Limited English proficiency has, in the past been shown to be a contributor to healthcare disparities (14) and is also likely to be a contributor in the context of EHRs and electronic media among affected populations unless appropriate accommodations in the information architecture are included in the EHR design.

2.6.3 People Living with Disabilities

According to the 2000 U.S. census, an estimated 19% (about 1 in 5) people in the United States have a disability (roughly 50 million people). Approximately 5.2 million (8%) were between the ages of 5 and 20. Another 30.6 million (57%) were between the ages of 21 and 64 and the remaining 14.0 million (42%) were 65 and over. This makes people with disabilities the largest minority in the country. It includes people who have disabilities that vary from mild to severe, and it includes people with temporary as well as chronic disabilities. The size of this demography is surprising to many people because of a limiting conception of people with disabilities as those with visual manifestations of their disability (e.g., you can see white canes, service dogs, sign language, and wheelchairs). In fact, many people with disabilities have an invisible impairment undetectable by simply looking at them (e.g., those who are hard of hearing) (61).

The Americans with Disabilities Act (ADA) of 1990 defines disability as the "inability to engage in any substantial gainful activity by reason of any medically determinable physical or mental impairment which can be expected to result in death or has lasted or can be expected to last for a continuous period of not less than 12 months" or "blindness" as defined as "central visual acuity of 20/200 or less in the better eye with the use of a correcting lens (62)."

The World Health Organization defines disabilities as follows: Disabilities is an umbrella term, covering impairments, activity limitations, and participation restrictions. An impairment is a problem in body function or structure; an activity limitation is a difficulty encountered by an individual in executing a task or action; while a participation restriction is a problem experienced by an individual in involvement in life situations. Thus disability is a complex phenomenon, reflecting an interaction between features of a person's body and features of the society in which he or she lives (63). As such, several types of disabilities which could impact EHR utilization and the outcomes are recognized by the ADA. These impairments could significantly impact the patients' and providers' ability to appropriately use and/or benefit from EHRs thus exacerbating illness, disease and potentially, disparities too. These impairments and their relationship to EHRs and healthcare disparities will be discussed below.

2.6.3.1 Hearing Impairment

In 2008, approximately 35 million people (11.3% of U.S. population) were hearing impaired. This number is expected to increase to approximately 40 million by 2050 (64). There are two major dimensions that have a large impact on the experience of hearing impairment: age of onset and severity of hearing loss. Combined, these two dimensions create several categories of hearing impairment. Age of onset includes 2 sets of persons. One includes persons who were deaf at birth or very early in infancy. This person has been deprived of the opportunity to acquire normal speech and language patterns, thus the problem in communication is linguistic as well as aural. The other includes persons in whom hearing impairment occurs after the acquisition of normal speech and language patterns. Included in this group are those whose hearing loss is the result of injury, illness, or old age. Problem in communication is aural rather than linguistic (65).

Hearing loss may minimally impact on EHR usability or healthcare disparities except for audible alerts. If an EHR system relies on audible alerts to communicate important information to users, the needs of hearing impaired users would not be adequately accommodated placing them at increased risk of usability problems and poorer health outcomes.

2.6.3.2 Physical Disability and Motor Impairment

Physical or mobility impairment is defined as a limitation in independent, purposeful physical movement of the body or of one or more extremities. The alteration in a person's mobility may be either temporary, or more permanent. Most of the diseases and rehabilitative states involved in physical and mobility impairments do involve a degree of immobility. These are often associated with things such as leg fractures, strokes, morbid obesity, trauma, and Multiple Sclerosis. As well, mobility is related to changes in a person's body as they age. Loss in muscle strength and mass, less mobile and stiffer joints, as well as gait changes affect a person's balance and may significantly comprise their mobility. Mobility is crucial to the maintenance of independent living among seniors. If a person's mobility is restricted, it may affect their activities of daily living (66). The major types of motor impairment and their implications for EHR usability and healthcare disparities will be discussed in the following sections.

2.6.3.2.1 Fine Motor Control Impairment

Fine motor skills involve the coordination of small muscle movements which occur usually in coordination with the eyes. Loss of fine motor control can make viewing and using an EHR more difficult for seniors and thus less likely that they will use the EHR system appropriately or at all. Most commonly seen among seniors, limitations in fine motor control may also occur in the context of many other diseases and health conditions leading to an increased risk of visual-perception problems. These may increase cognitive workload and limit information comprehension and understanding. It is also likely that a poorer user experience would inhibit EHR adoption. Research has demonstrated that improving the usability of systems by addressing fine motor control related to human factors issues will also allow all users to benefit from improved usability (9).

2.6.3.2.2 Dexterity Limitations

When referring to fine motor skills of the hands and fingers, the term dexterity is commonly used. Loss of dexterity is a common problem which puts afflicted individuals at increased risk of EHR related disparities because it can reduce the usability of EHR systems. Dexterity limitations therefore must be considered in EHR design if widespread usability is to be achieved particularly among seniors who have the highest prevalence of these limitations. Arthritis is very common in the US population and is a major cause of mobility, fine motor and dexterity limitations. Another common dexterity related condition is Parkinson's Disease. Parkinson's is a progressive condition affecting movements such as walking, talking, and writing (67). The four primary symptoms of Parkinson's Disease are tremors (trembling in the hands, arms, legs, jaw and face), rigidity (stiffness of the limbs and trunk), slowness of movement (bradykinesia) and impaired balance and coordination (67). Parkinson's Disease can also lead to cognitive and visual problems. Both arthritis and Parkinson's are likely to cause difficulties with the use of mouse, other pointing devices, and keyboard in some sufferers (67).

2.6.3.3 Visual Impairment

2.6.3.3.1 The Blind

There is no single universally accepted definition of blindness. The Americans with Disabilities Act defines "blindness" as "central visual acuity of 20/200 or less in the better eye with the use of a correcting lens (62), while the Social Security Administration considers one blind if either the best eye cannot be corrected to better than 20/200, or the visual field is less than or equal to

20 degrees with the aid of corrective lenses (62). The World Health Organization's (WHO) International Statistical Classification of Diseases and Related Health Problems (ICD-10) defines blindness as visual acuity of "less than 3/60 (0.05) or corresponding visual field loss in the better eye with best possible correction" (visual impairment categories 3, 4, and 5 in ICD-10). This corresponds to loss of walk-about vision. Finally, the U.S. Bureau of the Census simplifies its definition into lay terms as unable to see regular-sized newsprint (65).

Almost all U.S. government agencies have adopted the use of medical measurements broken down into three categories of visual impairment, which are used to determine eligibility for services and financial compensation: 1. Totally blind; 2. Legally blind (20/200 or less visual acuity in the best corrected eye {20/200 visual acuity means that what a fully sighted person sees from 200 feet away, a person with 20/200 vision sees from 20 feet away}, and/or 20 degrees or less in the visual field); 3. Partially sighted 20/70 visual acuity in the best corrected eye or 20 degrees or less in the visual field) (65). Individuals are legally blind when the best corrected central acuity is less than 20/200 (perfect visual acuity is 20/20) in your better eye, or your side vision is narrowed to 20 degrees or less in your better eye (68). People who are legally blind may still have some useful vision. Without appropriate EHR accommodation, visual problems will all lead to varying levels of visual-perception and associated cognitive and comprehension challenges among affected users,

2.6.3.3.2 Low Vision (Legally Blind)

Low vision is a term that denotes a level of vision that is 20/70 or worse and cannot be fully corrected with conventional glasses. Low vision is not the same as blindness. Vision loss that may be severe enough to impede a person's ability to carry on everyday activities, but still allows some functionally useful sight. Low vision may be caused by eye conditions or diseases. Low vision may range from moderate impairment to near-total blindness. It cannot be fully corrected by eyeglasses, contact lenses, or surgery. However, a person with low vision may benefit from any of a variety of available optical devices, such as electronic magnifying glasses or eyeglass-mounted telescopes. In addition, special computer software developed for patients and providers with low vision can display the type in large size or read text aloud (69).

2.6.3.3.3 Poor Vision (Not Legally Blind)

Vision impairment (poor vision) is vision loss to such a degree as to qualify for additional support through a significant limitation of visual capability resulting from either disease, trauma, or congenital or degenerative conditions that cannot be corrected by glasses, medication, or surgery. However the level of impairment is not such that it constitutes legal blindness. Common conditions associated with visual impairments include albinism, astigmatism, cataract, glaucoma, hyperopia, myopia, nystagmus, retinitis pigmentosa, retrolental fibroplasia (RLF) and strabismus (70).

2.6.3.3.4 Color Deficiencies including Color Blindness

Physically, color vision is defined by the response of the cone cells in the retina of the eye, which transform light into a set of three color responses, very much as a digital camera filters light to produce red, green, and blue pixel values. Statistically, people with normal color vision all have the same "normal" cone response though in practice there is some variation. People with a color vision deficiency have one or more cone responses that deviate significantly from normal. Perceptually, color is organized into three dimensions: hue, lightness, and colorfulness. Hue corresponds to the name of the color, such as red, green, or purple. Lightness is the perceived lightness of a color. Colorfulness, sometimes called saturation or chroma, indicates how vivid the color is (71). Approximately 8% of Caucasian males have a difficulty perceiving reds and greens. Abnormal response to blues, purples, and yellows is very rare genetically (less than 1%), but affects men and women equally. However, it can be caused by head injury, disease, or medication, especially in older viewers (71).

According to the American Foundation for the Blind, color blindness is a vision problem in which a person has difficulty distinguishing certain colors—most commonly red and green, but sometimes blue and green or blue and yellow. Color blindness is not really a form of blindness. Common problems associated with different forms of color vision deficiency include a) green will appear lighter and more yellowish. Green on white may be impossible to see. Green and amber will be difficult to distinguish. b) Red colors will appear darker, making red on black especially difficult to see. Brown and gray will be difficult to distinguish. c) Some people have difficulty distinguishing red from green, though those only mildly affected can do so if the colors are sufficiently strong. A less appreciated, but potentially more common problem is distinguishing colors that differ only by the addition of red or green, such as blue vs. purple, yellow vs. orange, blue vs. cyan (aqua, teal), and gray vs. brown. Certain individuals have difficulty distinguishing blue from green and yellow from purple while others can see only two hues distinct from gray, plus lightness variations. Finally a small percentage of people see only shades of gray. Many of these have other visual problems as well (lack of acuity, sensitivity to light) (71).

2.6.3.4 Psychological (Cognitive) Disability

The word "cognitive" refers to the functions of the brain: knowing, thinking and learning. Some people are born with cognitive disabilities, such as autism or mental retardation, which can hinder development. Other cognitive disabilities can be caused by traumatic brain injury or stroke, while others can result from diseases that develop later in life, such as Alzheimer's disease.

These can be associated with a host of medical and health problems including poor medication adherence (missed doses, over/under dosing, mixing/confusing medications), errors in judgment, poor healthcare decision making and inappropriate behaviorism. Many cognitive disabilities have a base in physiological or biological processes within the individual, such as a genetic disorder or a traumatic brain injury. Other cognitive disabilities may be based in the chemistry or structure of the person's brain. Persons with more profound cognitive disabilities often need assistance with aspects of daily living. Persons with minor learning disabilities might be able to function adequately despite their disability, maybe, to the point where their disability is never diagnosed or noticed (72).

Cognitive disability puts affected EHR users at increased risk of poor outcomes and healthcare disparities because it is associated with several problems like reading comprehension, communication (verbal and written) impairment, confusion and inappropriate EHR utilization. Sometimes it is more useful to avoid the medical perspective of cognitive disability and view them from a functional perspective. A functional disability perspective focuses on the abilities and challenges the person with a cognitive disability faces. Functional cognitive disabilities may involve problem-solving, attention, memory, and math, visual, reading, linguistic, and verbal comprehension (72).

Dyslexia is the most common form of language-based learning disability. Approximately fifteen to twenty percent of the population has some form of language-based learning disability. Dyslexia is primarily a reading disability, and there is evidence suggesting that dyslexia is a condition that is inherited. Dyslexia involves difficulty in single word decoding, often reflecting an insufficient phonological processing ability. This lack of ability is something that is many times unexpected in relation to the person's age and other cognitive and academic abilities. The person has not experienced another form of developmental disability, or sensory impairment. The person may have trouble with different forms of language, reading, and difficulty with spelling and writing as well (72).

Attention Deficit Hyperactivity Disorder (ADHD) is a medical condition affecting a person's ability to focus, sit still, and pay attention. Persons with ADHD may have difficulty in focusing on tasks or subjects, or act impulsively; they may also get into trouble. ADHD begins in childhood, but may not be diagnosed until the person reaches adolescence or even adulthood. Persons with ADHD may have difficulty with finishing assignments from school or tasks from home, jumping from one activity to another. They may lose things; forget things like homework or something they were supposed to do. They may have difficulty with following instructions, or following through with tasks they have been assigned. The person may make careless mistakes, or have difficulty paying attention to details. Persons with ADHD may have trouble organizing activities, or tasks, and may interrupt other people. They may fidget, feel restless, or talk excessively. Other major categories of functional cognitive disabilities include deficits or difficulties with memory, problem-solving, attention, reading, linguistic, and verbal comprehension, math comprehension and visual comprehension (72).

The main reason why these functional disabilities are more useful when considering EHR accessibility is that they are more directly related to the concerns of EHR developers. Telling a developer that some people have autism is not very meaningful unless the developer knows what kinds of barriers a person with autism might face. On the other hand, telling a developer that some people have difficulties comprehending math, provides the developer with a framework for addressing this type of audience (73).

Cognitive disability entails a substantial limitation in one's capacity to think, including conceptualizing, planning, sequencing thoughts and actions, remembering, interpreting subtle social cues, and understanding numbers and symbols. Cognitive disabilities include intellectual disabilities and can also stem from brain injury, Alzheimer's Disease and other dementias, severe and persistent mental illness, and, in some cases, stroke (73).

The definition used most often in the United States is that intellectual disability is a disability that occurs before age 18. It is characterized by significant limitations in intellectual functioning and adaptive behavior as expressed in conceptual, social and practical adaptive skills. Intellectual disabilities are also known as developmental delay or mental retardation. Intellectual functioning, also called intelligence, refers to general mental capacity, such as learning, reasoning, problem solving, etc. One criterion to measure intellectual functioning is an IQ test. Generally, an IQ test score of around 70 or as high as 75 indicates a limitation in intellectual functioning. But in defining and assessing intellectual disability, professionals must take additional factors into account, such as the community environment typical of the individual's peers and culture. Professionals should also consider linguistic diversity and cultural differences in the way people communicate, move, and behave (73). Finally, assessments must also assume that limitations in individuals often coexist with strengths, and that a person's level of life functioning will improve if appropriate personalized supports are provided over a sustained period (73).

2.6.4 Seniors and the Elderly

In 2000, there were 281.4 million people in the United States. Approximately 72 million (26 %) were under age 18, 174.1 million (62%) were age 18 to 64 and 35.0 million (12%) were over the age of 65. The median age of the U.S. population increased from 32.9 in 1990 to 35.3 in 2000. Also in 2000, the two largest 5-year age groups were 35-to-39 year olds with 22.7 million people (8.1% of the total population) and 40-to-44 year olds with 22.4 million people (8.0% of the population). People in these two age groups were primarily born during the post-World War II "Baby Boom" (those born from 1946 through 1964). In Census 2000, the baby boom cohort was age 36 to 54 and represented 28 percent of the total U.S. population (74).

In terms of rate of growth the 50-to-54 year old age group experienced a 55% growth in population over the past decade while 45-to-49 age group experienced a 45% increase. The baby-boom cohort entered these two age groups during the past decade. The third fastest-growing group in the past decade was 90-to-94-year olds, which increased by 45%. On the other hand four age groups declined over the past decade. These include the 25-to-29 year olds (9% decrease), 30-to-34 year olds (6% decrease), 65-to-69 year olds (6% decrease), and 20-to-24 year olds (0.3% decrease). The number of people in the younger age groups, especially those aged 25 to 34, fell as the baby boom cohort aged into older age groups. The decline in 65-to-69 year olds is associated with a relatively low number of births during the early 1930s (74).

Seniors are a target population at increased risk for experiencing healthcare disparities with EHR use because increasing age is often accompanied by increasing levels of human factors challenges that may impact EHR usability. The commonly accepted limitations that often arise during the normal aging process, which may impact EHR usability, include vision decline, hearing loss, motor skill diminishment and cognitive effects. (See section 2.6.3) In addition the aging process can often result in elderly people experiencing multiple functional limitations. Each of these major areas will be briefly described below.

2.6.4.1 Age-Related Vision Decline

A variety of vision changes may occur with aging. These include decreasing ability to focus on near tasks, including a computer screen and color perception and sensitivity problems causing less violet light to be registered (67). This has the effect of making it easier to see red and yellows than blues and greens and often making darker blues and black indistinguishable. In addition seniors often have pupil shrinkage resulting in the need for more light and a diminished capacity to adjust to changing light levels (67). They also suffer contrast sensitivity loss. In fact, from the age of 40, contrast sensitivity at higher spatial frequencies starts to decline until at the age of 80 when it has been shown to be reduced by up to 83% (67). Reduction in visual field is another vision problem associated with aging that can seriously affect vision. Visual field loss can be caused by Cataracts which is a treatable disease resulting in a clouding of the clear lens in the eye, causing blurred vision and glare sensitivity (67). Visual field loss may also be caused by what is known as Age-related Macular Degeneration (AMD). AMD is incurable and results in central vision deterioration and an inability to see fine detail and distinguish color possibly combined with a sensitivity to glare (67).

2.6.4.2 Age-Related Hearing Loss

In terms of hearing loss, seniors often notice a gradual age-related reduction and the increasing inability to hear high pitched sounds. It is estimated that around the age of 50 the proportion of deaf people begins to increase sharply and 55% of people over 60 are deaf or hard of hearing (67).

2.6.4.3 Age-Related Cognitive Decline

The ability to encode new memories of events or facts and working memory show declines in both cross-sectional and longitudinal studies (75). Studies comparing the effects of aging on episodic memory, semantic memory, short-term memory and priming find that episodic memory is especially impaired in normal aging (76). These deficits may be related to impairments seen in the ability to refresh recently processed information (77). In addition, even when equated in memory for a particular item or fact, older adults tend to be worse at remembering the source of their information (78), a deficit that may be related to declines in the ability to bind information together in memory (79). It has also been suggested that situation awareness may be relevant to cognitive aging, affecting older adults' perception and comprehension of their environment (80).

While most older adults may not suffer from dementia or Alzheimer's Disease, many do suffer Mild Cognitive Impairment (MCI) or subjective memory loss (67). The issues associated with MCI include trouble remembering the names of people, trouble remembering the flow of a conversation and an increased tendency to misplace things. All these complaints are likely to also impact on the use of EHRs (67).

2.6.5 Racial and Ethnic Minorities

Racial and ethnic minorities have been shown to be at increased risk for Healthcare disparities. Despite many differences, as a group they also share some characteristics that may have human factors implications for the design, adoption and utilization of EHR systems. For example, racial and ethnic minorities are more likely to speak a non-English language as their primary language used in the home. As such, understanding even simple English words and phrases may prove challenging. They are also at higher risk of having limited English proficiency. They are also more likely to receive care from a healthcare safety net provider working in a low resource setting with a user context significantly different from that of another provider working in an alternate setting. Finally, racial and ethnic minorities are more likely to have mental models of health and illness that differ from those of a healthcare provider born and trained in the United States. These other models include beliefs that health/illness is ordained by God, and choices about healthcare service utilization are made in a communal fashion only after discussion with other respected members of the group. Attempting to facilitate patient healthcare decisions via use of the EHR may lead to patients intentionally providing erroneous or misleading information, failing to utilize or underutilizing the EHR system because of lack of trust or in an effort to avoid culturally difficult situations. All of these could potentially impact patient outcomes among this user group.

3   EHR Technical Considerations of Healthcare Disparities

The following sections present an overview of those steps in the EHR design process that potentially impact healthcare disparities. Current vendor practices indicate that EHR design and development strategies only minimally consider formal Human Factors Engineering (HFE) and ergonomics design principles if at all (7). As such, there may be an under appreciation of the potential magnitude of the impact of design flaws on usability and the context of use that could lead to healthcare disparities.

3.1.1   The EHR Development Life Cycle

The EHR design process shall be an iterative process that involves: 1) planning and development of EHR requirements and specifications; 2) designing and building the EHR to planned specifications; and 3) review and testing of the EHR prototype. An optimal EHR is the product of multiple development, design, prototyping, review and evaluation iterations. In addition, early involvement of users in development is an absolute requirement to the development of high quality and usable EHRs.

In terms of healthcare disparities, there is no evidence that involvement of a reasonable set of representative users (providers, patients, caregivers) from disparity populations are consistently involved in all phases of the design process. As such, current EHR designs may not adequately meet the needs, provide optimal user experiences or be appropriately usable by all providers (aging providers, providers with disabilities) caring for patients at increased risk of disparities or among patients and caregivers from disparity populations. The EHR design and development considerations most likely to impact the risk of healthcare disparities will be briefly outlined below (81).

3.1.1.1   EHR Planning

The EHR planning process consists of preparing a complete and comprehensive design and development plan for all intended EHR users. The plan is based on the articulation of clear design requirements for each type of user, all user tasks and each type of user environment. Essential EHR design requirements that may impact healthcare disparities include task analysis, user experience requirements, EHR interface design requirements, user living and working condition (user context) and cultural requirements (81). Failure to adequately consider these design elements could lead to a reliance on inappropriate or incorrect design assumptions regarding a given type of EHR user or user context.

3.1.1.1.1   Task Analysis

A task analysis is the collection and analysis of information about the intended users of the system and the tasks that they will perform. The design requirements should be based on comprehensive task analyses. An overall concept should be developed of the users (providers, support staff, patients' caregivers, etc.), their needs and their roles in managing health and healthcare tasks. The effect of the EHR on the existing tasks of individual users should be analyzed. This should include a consideration of any potential changes that may result from the initial combined use of electronic and paper-based systems. The effects of the EHR system on user communications should be evaluated. Tasks should be analyzed and used as an input to design. Tasks associated with failure and backup should be identified to define the requirement for indicating malfunctions. The task of smoothly transitioning from a paper based system to an EHR system and back to a back-up paper system, if needed, in the event of system failure, all should be explicitly analyzed and addressed (82).

EHRs should be designed to take account of the people who will use them. Therefore, all relevant user groups should be identified. Constructing systems based on an inappropriate or incomplete understanding of user needs is one of the major sources of systems failure. It is likely also to be a potential contributor to the development of healthcare disparities. The extent to which products are usable and accessible depends on the context of use. The characteristics of the patients and providers, tasks and environment in which the EHRs will be used, comprise the context of use (17). The context of use is a major source of information for establishing requirements and an essential input to the design process (17). Provider, patient and caregiver user contexts will not always be the same. Patient and provider contexts may be the same during a clinical encounter; however, it is likely that, in the future, patients will increasingly interact with their providers and EHRs in both synchronous (in real time) and asynchronous (via messaging) fashion in the context of both face to face and remote clinical encounters. Given this reality, the steps required to accomplish a given task or even the required tasks needed to accomplish a given function may themselves differ depending on the context in which the patient may be using (e.g., home) vs. that in which the provider may be using (e.g., clinic or Emergency Department). Assumptions about patient and caregiver user contexts based on provider user contexts will likely lead to inadequate designs. In addition, the user contexts between different types of providers (safety net providers, academic clinicians, rural solo practitioners) may be sufficiently different that inadequate attention to this issue could lead to poor designs for one or more types of providers. As can be seen, robust task analysis among all intended users is a critical determinant of usable EHRs that do not contribute to healthcare disparities. (82)

Task analyses should also identify the implications of working conditions requiring competing demands on attention and mental workload of users. The basis for these analyses can be found in Multiple Resource Theory (83). It is imperative that designers have an explicit understanding of the EHR user contexts in order to be able to accurately distinguish compatible tasks (those which can be safely performed simultaneously) from incompatible tasks (those which carry a higher risk of error, data loss or other harm, if performed simultaneously). With this knowledge, EHR system architects can better design systems that support provider or patient focal tasks (the task judged to be most important) without causing inappropriate task incompatibility or forcing an EHR user to focus attention on a less important task (distracter) because of system design defects (83).

Finally, task analyses should also provide a basis for determining training requirements for all EHR users (82). The training program should address the role of the providers and patients to assure that they remain in control of the EHR system. The knowledge, skills, and abilities that patients and providers will require to interact successfully with the EHR should be specified by the designers (82). Computer/technology literacy, computer familiarity and technology related user anxiety have all been shown to be health IT usability barriers among the elderly, chronically ill, disabled and medically underserved patients (84;85). On the other hand, computer training, technology support and lost productivity due to prolonged training have all been implicated as usability and adoption barriers among providers, especially those caring for the nation's most vulnerable patients (86;87).

3.1.1.1.2 User Experience requirements

User experience is defined as a person's perceptions and responses resulting from the use and/or anticipated use of a product, system or service (17). Usability can be seen as one aspect of the total user experience. On the other hand, poor user experience with a technology may inhibit usability and adoption. The EHR user experience then, is a consequence of several factors including the presentation, functionality, system performance, interactive behavior, and assistive capabilities of the system. It has been shown to impact beliefs about ease of use and perceived usefulness (88). Minority providers, solo practitioners and providers caring for underserved populations often report lack of perceived usefulness of EHRs as a significant barrier to adoption and utilization. Thus, among those providers most likely to care for patients from disparity populations, lack of attention to user experience when designing EHRs could facilitate EHR adoption disparities. To effectively reduce healthcare disparities it may prove important to determine the user experience requirements for patients and caregivers. If EHRs are designed to provide optimal user experience for the providers, they may fail to provide the same for patients and contribute to poor patient utilization of EHRs despite provider utilization. Important considerations that may impact user experience will be briefly discussed below.

3.1.1.1.3 User Living Environment (Context) Requirements

The extent to which EHRs are usable and accessible depends in part on the physical environment in which they will be used. The relevant characteristics of the environment that impact usability must be described for each user context. Important physical attributes include issues such as thermal conditions, lighting, spatial layout and furniture. Currently, there is substantial ongoing effort to understand these issues in the hospital, clinic or practice environment.

For example, it is well known that among individuals living in rural America, access to primary care is a significant challenge. Approximately one quarter of the U.S. population lives in rural America yet only 10% of all physicians live and practice in these areas (89). The obstacles faced by healthcare providers and patients in rural areas are, at times, vastly different than those in other areas. Rural Americans face a combination of factors that place them at increased risk of experiencing disparities in healthcare. Economic factors, cultural and social differences, educational shortcomings and the sheer isolation of living in remote rural areas all conspire to impede rural Americans in their struggle to lead a normal, healthy life as compared to those living in other environments (90).

In terms of EHRs and usability, EHR use is less common in rural locations and in small practices where access to broadband services are limited (91). The home and living environments of rural Americans likely present other important usability challenges that must be addressed. For similar reasons, the EHR accessibility, usability, lighting, humidity, safety and privacy issues associated with urban inner city and low income housing must be taken into consideration when developing EHRs for use by patients living in these settings.

3.1.1.1.4 Cultural Requirements

Historically, ergonomics as a discipline was started in North America and Western Europe and produced findings and data that apply primarily and best to Western customs, habits and ways of life (92). Increasingly though, culturally related problems with the interaction between users and technology are being attributed to lack of consideration of human factors (92).

Several aspects of culture have been evaluated by human factors and ergonomics experts and found to be of importance to interface design and usability. This field of study, called Cultural Ergonomics (CE), has mainly focused on applications in aviation and international user interfaces. CE does not argue that biological differences associated with membership in specific cultural groups accounts for differences in usability or behavior, but rather proposes that culture is a persistent situational phenomenon that is manifested through persistent patterns of interaction with the environment. These persistent patterns in behavior directly extend from beliefs, values, and mental models. Thus, cultural influences are environmental, and therefore, situation-based (93).

Given the substantial racial and ethnic demographic shifts occurring in the US, the implications of existing differences in health paradigms or mental models of health across patient populations will, at a minimum, require EHR accommodations based on appropriate use case data. In "Western" countries, the allopathic or "orthodox" medical model is the dominant health paradigm. However, there are also two other models of Western healthcare, the social model and the psychological model. These models have different assumptions about the nature of illness and wellness and differences of approach to the maintenance of good health and the treatment of illness. They also often use different terms for the same health concept (e.g. "problems" in the medical model and "issues" in the social model). However, differences between Western and non-Western health models are generally greater than those between the three Western models (94).

Oriental medicine (e.g. Chinese medicine) and Ayurvedic medicine, collectively often called "alternative" or "complementary" medicine in Western countries, are fundamentally different from Western orthodox medicine. The practitioners of these different health models not only use different terms for the same entity but sometimes also use the same term to express different concepts. For example, the terms "inflammation" and "elevated calcium" have quite different meanings for Western and some alternative/complementary practitioners (94).

A single EHR, across different health paradigms, could be very beneficial for the holistic care of patients seeking care from practitioners of different health models (estimated to be more than 50% of the population in many countries). However, it could also be potentially dangerous or even life-threatening for a patient, unless different technical assumptions and different meanings for the same terms are recognized and incorporated into the EHR (94). There is little, if any, experience as yet, in using a single EHR across different health paradigms but there are techniques available in the evolving model-based EHR standards to assist in dealing with these challenges. For example, the use of "folders" within the EHR is one way to segregate different types of EHR content. Also different folders may be used for acute hospital care, primary care, mental health, and "alternative" care practitioners such as herbalists and naturopaths. The use of archetypes for clinical content and distinct domain-specific term sets to underpin the archetypes will also assist in avoiding problems due to different healthcare paradigms within a single EHR (94).

3.1.1.1.5 EHR Human-Computer Interface Requirements

Among providers, the organization and display of information is essential to effectively support clinical care, maximizing usability and reducing the potential for user error (95). The EHR user interface, through which the care team enters and retrieves patient information, care guidelines and medical evidence must be highly efficient, intuitive, and responsive to varying clinical information needs, to adequately support the practice of medicine (95). Because EHRs will also support doctor-patient communication, patient education and enhance patient engagement in disease management, the interface must also support the needs of patients and caregivers.

There are at least 2 key factors that can impact interface requirements that may affect healthcare disparities with the use of EHRs. These are the role of disability (See section 2.6.3) and culture (See Section 2.7.1.3) on the information architecture. It is likely that these factors will predominately affect patient and caregiver EHR usability. However, to the extent that providers are themselves becoming an increasingly diverse population, these factors may also have some impact on provider EHR usability. The existing research and knowledge regarding the role of culture specifically on interface design and usability will be outlined below.

Almost 3 decades ago cultural differences in everything from the legibility of alphabetic characters (96), to working posture were described and explored for the implications of these differences on design. More recently, it has been shown that cultural factors influence appropriate mappings between controls and displays (97), colors and concepts (98) and icons and concepts (99). For example, while 100% of Americans associated the concept stop with the color red, only 48.5% of Chinese agreed with this mapping. Additional work in this domain has shown that there are cultural differences in the appropriate navigational structure (100;101) and the type of overarching metaphor used in computer displays (102). In the 1990s, the concept of "hidden cultural assumptions" (103) in health information technology was put forth which suggested that although designers often believe their creations are culturally neutral, in actuality, technologies embody cultural assumptions that may not always be appropriate for the intended user.

EHR user characteristics which exhibit cultural variability can be grouped into two basic categories. These include physical characteristics and visual/cognitive characteristics. Physical characteristics or anthropometry, from an engineering standpoint, is concerned with integrating physical characteristics into the development of engineering design standards (92) However, applying American anthropometric design standards without any adjustment to other populations of the world may cause significant problems. In general, an interface design which is suitable to fit 95% of Americans, fits 90% of Germans, 80% of the French population, 65% of Indian population, 45% of the Japanese, 25% of Thais and only 10% of Vietnamese (92). The implications of such variations for technology design problems and the degree of required changes and/or adjustments that may be needed are significant. Consideration has to be given not only to display height, but also sitting statures, working postures, and leg length in proportion to height. It has been convincingly shown that simply scaling up or down to fit these anthropometric differences simply does not work (92).

Studies of perceptual processes have shown that perception has cultural characteristics with regard to interpretation of observations and data. For example, Nepalese individuals have significant difficulty reading and interpreting maps and spatially oriented diagrams while Vietnamese individuals have difficulty understanding and interpreting technical drawings (92). Research evaluating preferences in direction-of-movement tendencies found that strong direction of movement preferences exist in Western culture (read from left to right, off = turning dials left to right, on = turning dials right to left, etc). Subjects of individuals of non-western ethnicity and nationality indicate that these preferences are not universally held and are subject to local exposure and education (92).

The mental processes of different cultures may also impact usability of EHRs. This is because differences in performance levels of individuals of different cultural backgrounds is not usually caused by differences in cognitive capabilities of the individuals rather the primary factors responsible for observed differences are individuals' cognitive complexity, information processing behavior, and psychomotor skill (92). The potential for developing complex cognitive abilities exists; it merely needs to be stimulated and exercised through application of appropriate training procedures. Cognitive characteristics and perceptual processes, therefore, are culturally influenced. Awareness of the potential influence on the performance of a particular task or usability of a given tool is necessary and should be made a major consideration in determining the human-computer interface requirements for future EHRs.

Finally, objective evidence exists suggesting a link between culture and usability (104). Some cultural dimensions including power distance, individualism versus collectivism, and uncertainty avoidance may impact usability and may be affected by user interface design (104). Power distance measures the extent to which the less powerful members of a group accept and expect that power is distributed unequally. Low power distance scores reflect less acceptance of the unequal distribution of power, while higher scores reflect greater acceptance of unequal distribution of power within one's culture (104). Individualism and collectivism focuses on the relationship between the individual and groups. Highly individualistic cultures (European) believe that the individual is the most important unit while highly collectivistic cultures (Asian, African-American) believe that the group is the most important unit. Low scores indicate strong collectivism while high scores suggest strong individualism within a given culture (104). Finally, Uncertainty Avoidance (UA) is the extent to which a culture feels threatened or anxious about ambiguity and how hard individuals will work to avoid it. UA focuses on how cultures adapt to change and cope with uncertainty. As such, low UA cultures tend to respond well to ambiguity and uncertainty while high UA cultures do not (104).

Patients who exhibit high uncertainty avoidance may experience greater frustration with certain interface designs (104). In addition, individuals from cultures with low power distance indicators (e.g., people more accepting of uneven power distribution) may be more likely to score higher on usability testing of an interface than individuals from cultures with high power distance indicators (104).

3.1.2 The Potential of EHR Technical Design Issues to Impact Healthcare Disparities

As can be seen from the above discussion, there are potentially many opportunities during the EHR design and development lifecycle, where oversights, flawed designs or otherwise poor designs, based on faulty assumptions, lack of representative data or inadequate information architecture could contribute to reductions in EHR access, usability or adoption and in turn increase the risk of poor outcomes and healthcare disparities among at risk patient populations.

4   Technical Guidance and Recommendations

There is great need for federal coordination and integration across multiple agencies. Coordination must be built on explicit plans and strategies (105). One critical area of needed federal leadership is in the area of technical guidelines and standards that will help ensure broad accessibility and usability and thereby reduce the possibility of creating or exacerbating healthcare disparities with the roll out, adoption and utilization of EHRs and other emerging health IT products.

Because improvements in accessibility and usability tend to benefit everyone, addressing human factors challenges will likely benefit all EHR users. Improvements in EHR accessibility and usability will contribute to higher adoption rates among providers. Increasing meaningful use by providers combined with improving patient engagement in their healthcare through EHRs, will lead to improvements in healthcare quality and health outcomes. In addition, among patients with disabilities, those with limited English proficiency, lower socio demographic groups, and seniors, these improvements will likely also contribute to reductions in healthcare disparities. The following is a discussion of specific guidelines and recommendations that may be taken to reduce the risk of healthcare disparities on healthcare delivery with the adoption of EHRs.

4.1   EHR Design and Development Guidelines

Several design enhancements may significantly reduce the likelihood of introducing or exacerbating healthcare disparities with the adoption of EHRs. Generally, these recommendations focus on equipping the EHR design team with the necessary information needed to understand potential healthcare disparities challenges related to provider and patient use of the EHR. These recommendations also focus on ensuring that this information is then used to improve the iterative design process and ultimately make the appropriate product enhancements.

4.1.1 Conduct Comprehensive Formative and Summative Testing with a Reasonable Set of Representative End Users

To help ensure EHR accessibility and usability, it is imperative that developmental testing involve those who are likely to be using the system. While current EHR systems are designed primarily to facilitate medical practice by healthcare practitioners, they are intended to also be used to enhance physician-patient communication and engagement primarily in the context of a clinical encounter. As such, the needs of the patients and caregivers who will be interacting with the provider must be taken into consideration, if the information provided to the patient is to be understood and then used by the patient in shared decision making and disease self-management. Patients, consumers and caregivers, like providers, have a spectrum of physical, cognitive and other needs that can significantly affect physician-patient communication, understanding, motivation and ultimately outcomes. A large body of human factors research has been done regarding human-computer interactions and accommodations. Many technical accommodations have been developed, tested and validated as effective in addressing potential human factors needs. This body of knowledge should be integrated into the design of current and emerging EHR systems, to ensure the widest possible accessibility and usability and to ensure the safe, effective and error free interactions with EHRs by the end users. The importance of considering the needs of providers must not be ignored nor underappreciated.

However, considering only the needs of the provider will tend to minimize the physician's ability to provide consistent, high quality, patient-centered care and improve patient health outcomes.

4.1.2 Report Results of the Tests in Common Industry Format (CIF) for EHR Usability Test Reports

Usability of EHR systems is a key factor in predicting successful deployment. EHR system developers must subject EHRs to usability testing at various stages in a product's development cycle. Testing should involve (1) test participants who are representative of the target population of EHR users, (2) representative tasks, and (3) measures of efficiency, effectiveness and subjective satisfaction. The Common Industry Format (CIF) is intended for reporting the results of usability testing (8).

Given the plethora of EHR products and vendors, CIF is valuable because it standardizes the types of information that should be captured regarding testing with users. The major variables include user demographics, task descriptions, context of the test, including the equipment used, the environment in which the test is conducted and the protocol by which the subjects and the test administrator(s) interact, as well as the particular metrics chosen to code the findings of the study. The CIF is intended to replace proprietary formats employed by EHR vendors, developers and purchasers that perform usability testing. The advantages of using a standardized reporting format include (1) a reduction in training time for usability staff since an individual only needs to learn to use one and (2) enhanced potential for increased communication between vendors and purchasing organizations since readers of CIF-compliant reports will share a common language and expectations.

Another purpose of the CIF is to facilitate incorporation of usability testing into the procurement decision-making process for EHR systems so that it is easier to judge whether a product meets the usability goals. It provides a common format to report the methods and results of usability tests to customer organizations (8).

CIF should be used by usability professionals within supplier organizations to generate reports that can be used by customer organizations. The CIF is also meant to be used by customer organizations to verify that a particular report is CIF-compliant. As such, the usability test report itself is intended for two types of readers: 1) Usability professionals in customer organizations who are evaluating both the technical merit of usability tests and the usability of the products; and 2) Other technical professionals and managers who are using the test results to make business decisions. The CIF may also be used within a single organization if a formal report of a summative usability test needs to be generated. In this case additional material such as a list of detailed findings may be included (8).

4.1.3 Accommodate as Many EHR Users as Possible Using Universal Design Principles

To ensure that as many users as possible including safety net providers practicing in under resourced settings and patients from disparities populations are able to safely and effectively use emerging EHR systems, a universal design strategy should be adopted. Universal design principles incorporate user-centered design, universal usability and universal accessibility principles to bring attention to both the potential EHR user challenges and accommodation solutions that might be otherwise overlooked. Accommodating a broader spectrum of users and user contexts will require designers to consider a wide range of designs. Many of the design accommodations can be incorporated without significant impact on developmental time or expense. Once completed, these improvements often lead to innovations that benefit all users (9). These features should include Graphic User Interface (GUI) elements that will support system novice users and at the same time will offer shortcuts to expert and advanced system users.

4.1.4 Include Disparities Oriented Use Cases as Part of the EHR Design and Development Process

EHR developers should use disparities oriented use case scenarios and user contexts to test how well their systems support providers caring for disparity populations. Incorporating such focused use-cases into the formative EHR development process could help developers overcome current expertise shortages and barriers to adoption and use by these providers.

Examples of disparities oriented use cases include:

1) **Safety net provider use case.** Developing and applying use cases involving common tasks specific to clinical practice in safety net contexts will be a key to elucidating unrecognized user requirements.

2) **Adult caregiver of a senior relative use case.** In many families, adult children caring for elderly parents, is becoming increasingly common. This may be even more likely among patients from disparity populations who may lack resources to provide alternate care arrangements for their aging relative. The cognitive and physical demands and stress of care giving combined with childrearing, homemaking and also additional employment may create human factors challenges for the safe and effective use of EHRs. In other words, the consideration of these broader patient user contexts, may be as critical for understanding EHR usability by patients as understanding clinical workflows in the hospital is for understanding provider EHR usability

3) **Patient/caregiver with limited English proficiency use case.** Providing care to patients with limited English proficiency creates challenges for all involved parties. This is no less true in the context of EHR mediated care. If patients cannot understand their English speaking healthcare providers they are not likely to understand their English language based EHRs. This is not surprising. What is less clear is what, if anything, these patients may do to overcome deficiencies of understanding, especially in the absence of appropriate accommodations when attempting to use, or access an EHR. Misunderstandings or confusion caused by a poorly designed EHR, in the context of marginal English proficiency may prove more challenging and more difficult to even detect than complete inability to use the available system unless these types of use cases are employed. Use plain language instructions to accommodate these user contingents.

4) **EHR use in the context of cross cultural or communications barriers use case.** In some cultures, major decision making, is considered a family or at least a combined activity between a husband and a wife. However, informed consent and access to EHR information is currently considered largely from the Western perspective (i.e. single users and individual rights). Usability, user experience and satisfaction implications with the use of such an EHR are not likely to be optimal. There may be design accommodations that could help address the challenges created by these cultural differences.

4.2 EHR Evaluation Guidelines

4.2.1 Require Documentation of Formative and Summative Testing with a Reasonable Set of Representative Target Users as a Prerequisite for EHR Evaluation

To ensure that appropriate formative and summative testing is indeed occurring, it is recommended that periodic documentation be provided as a part of the EHR evaluation and reevaluation process.

4.2.2 Require Documentation of Product Features Designed to Increase Usability and Accessibility or Documentation of a Lack of Need for any Accommodation among a Reasonable Set of Target Users

To ensure that vendors are making appropriate design enhancements specifically for the purpose of improving identified limitations among target users, it is recommended that documentation of included product features be provided as part of EHR evaluation and reevaluation process.

4.2.3 Require the Development of EHR Operation, Safety, Customer Support and Educational Materials that are Culturally and Linguistically Appropriate for a Reasonable Set of Representative Target Users as a Prerequisite for EHR Evaluation Process

Writing clear EHR related system messages and instructional and educational materials is critically important as an increasing variety of users adopts EHRs. The following specific recommendations are made for instructional materials for both paper and electronic formats (10). These should not be viewed as an exhaustive nor comprehensive set of recommendations. Rather these can be considered as a starting point for the development of more effective and usable EHR instructional materials.

EHR Operation and Safety Instructions Development Recommendations

1) **Put instructions where (at specific point on the screen) they are needed – not all together at the top of the page.** Instructions must come "just in time" – when EHR users need them – at the beginning of the section where they are relevant. Having all the instructions at the beginning, poses a heavy burden on EHR user's memory. People tend to pay attention only if the instructions seem relevant to their current needs. They may not read instructions that do not apply at the moment they are reading them. The more there is to read in one place, the more likely it is that many providers and clinicians will just skip the instructions. When instructions come "just in time," there are fewer to give at any one place (10).

2) **Put instructions above/before they are needed – not after** Instructions for specific parts of an EHR system must come just before the provider has to act. This guideline does not conflict with the previous one. Clinicians need instructions at the place in the EHR where the instruction is relevant. And they need those instructions just before and not after the options the instructions relate to. This is necessary because people read and act in the order in which information comes to them. They do not skip over the action part to look for instructions (10).

3) **Put instructions in logical order first task, first; last task, last.** Instructions for specific parts of an EHR must come in the order that providers and patients need them because they make more sense if they come in the order in which they will be used. Also, if providers have to go back to look for what to do in case of a problem, they will likely look to the end of a list of instructions (10).

4) **Put warnings about consequences before – not after – the provider is likely to act.** Providers and clinical staff must learn about the potential negative consequences of an action before the instruction to take the necessary action since people often act as soon as they see an instruction. If they act before reading the warning, they will not be able to heed the warning (10).

5) **Do not highlight the action option until providers have been given all available options.** Providers must be given all available options to choose from *before* they are given the signal to make the choice. This is because people are drawn to the first and brightest message they see. Flashing words or buttons are very eye-catching even when they are in peripheral vision. If a bright or flashing message suggests that it is time to take an action, many clinicians will be distracted and not realize that they have not yet looked at the rest of the screen (10).

6) **The order of buttons must match the order of the instructions.** The order of choices in the instructions and the order of the buttons that relate to those choices must match. Clinical staff may assume that the order is the same and inconsistency between the instruction and the buttons may cause some clinicians to make errors (10).

7) **Start each instruction on a new line.** Each instruction must start on a new line. Different instructions must not be combined together in a single paragraph. If each instruction starts on its own line, providers and clinical staff will be less likely to miss an instruction, can more easily see that there are multiple situations and multiple instructions and will more easily find an instruction if they come back to look for it. Under the time stress, busy clinicians often scan rather than read. Instructions on separate lines are easier to scan than instructions in a paragraph (10).

8) **Write directly to the clinician.** Instructions must be in the imperative (i.e., "Do this..."). Statements of fact or law must not replace instructions. Instructions tell people what to do. People are more likely to act appropriately when they read instructions than when they read statements about facts. Also, sentences with imperative verbs are in the active voice. English sentences can be in either active voice or passive voice. Passive sentences are more difficult to understand than active sentences because the pieces of a passive sentence are not in logical order from the clinicians' point of view (10).

9) **Keep each instruction as short as possible.** Instructions should be as short as while conveying the essential message. Leave out unnecessary words. Try to keep sentences to 20 words or less. Providers are more likely to read short sentences. Short sentences are also easier to remember (10).

10) **Watch the tone. Help clinicians, don't threaten them.** Often instructions tell providers, clinical staff or patients what to do if they somehow make an error and need to start again. The message about this must not blame the user. It must be in words that are clear to clinicians. It must have a friendly tone. individuals who feel blamed or shamed are less likely to make the necessary corrections (10).

11) **Write in the positive.** EHR instructions must be in the positive whenever possible. Rewrite double negatives as positive sentences because positive sentences are easier to understand. In English, two negatives make a positive. You can rewrite an English sentence that has two negatives into a simpler positive sentence (10).

12) **Put the context before the action.** Many instructions are sentences with two parts: a) what the user wants to do (the context, "to do...") and b) what the EHR user must do to accomplish that (the action, "do..."). EHR instructions must put the context before the action because research shows that if you give people the action before the context,

many will begin to act before reading the end of the sentence. Errors will be made because they did not read all of the instruction (10).

13) **Be consistent in the language of the instructions.** EHR instructions must keep the same pattern for similar instructions because providers are very pattern-oriented. Patterns help people grasp information quickly and accurately (10).

14) **Do not use gender-based pronouns.** Instructions and statements that are addressed to both men and women must not use references to only one or the other gender. If the statement refers to a particular person, it is correct to use the appropriate gender pronoun for that person. Gender-based pronouns and words exclude the other gender from consideration in the mind of the EHR user (10).

15) **Use simple English words.** The words used in EHR systems must be the ones that clinicians understand. While all clinicians have achieved a certain level of training and mastery of the English language, they also come from many ethnic and cultural backgrounds which can impact understanding or translation of difficult, compound, complex or obscure words or words without direct translations in the providers native language (10).

16) **Be consistent in the language that is used.** Instructions and messages must use words consistently. Once you name something, use that name throughout the EHR system. Providers may be confused if the same object has different names and they may think that the instructions and messages are talking about different objects (10).

17) **Do not use technical, computer jargon.** This is a special case of the guideline to use words clinicians know. Instructions and all other material must talk to clinicians in their language and not use technical, computer words that they are likely not to know. Many clinicians are not familiar with computer terminology. If they do not understand the instructions, they may act incorrectly, and require increased time to find out what to do which will decrease efficiency, productivity (10).

18) **Be explicit in naming buttons.** This is another special case of using appropriate words and using simple English. Buttons must be meaningful to providers. Touching or otherwise selecting buttons on EHRs are one way that providers take actions. They must understand what they are choosing with each button (10).

19) **Cover all important situations.** Although we do not want to overburden providers with instructions, they must have instructions for relevant situations. Where there are no instructions, there is an implicit assumption that clinicians will know what to do by themselves. If that assumption is wrong, some providers will be confused and errors may occur (10).

20) **Consider clinicians likely mistakes.** Instruction writers must think about the ways that busy clinicians might misinterpret the instructions. They must write instructions to avoid those misinterpretations. People always bring their earlier experiences to new situations. They have expectations from those earlier experiences that may make them interpret situations differently from the way that is intended (10).

Guidelines for designing clear EHR system messages

1) **Understand the audience for messages about problems.** On EHR systems, in addition to instructions and messages that clinicians see in the normal course of using the system, messages must be available for times when something goes wrong. It is imperative to understand the audience for messages about problems. The concern is for

any message that might be seen by a clinician. If the message could come up while a provider is using the EHR, the message must be clear to providers. If a message could come up while a clinical staff person, student or patient is using the system, the message must be clear to them. EHR users span a very wide range of literacy, of English language skills, and of experience with computers. Many users (providers or patients) are older people who did not grow up with computers or have never used computers.

2) **Understand the context for messages about problems.** It is important to understand the context for messages about problems. Troubleshooting messages appear only when the problem occurs. If a message comes up while a provider is trying to use the EHR it will almost certainly come as a surprise. The provider may have never seen the message before. Just seeing the message will be a source of stress and anxiety. These are all reasons why messages must be extremely clear, instantly understandable, include information on what to do, and be calming rather than blaming. All of these points are equally true for other clinical staff members, patients and caregivers who may also use the EHR. System messages can be greatly improved by following the following seven guidelines. 1) Do not call system messages "error messages". 2) Do not blame the user. 3) Explain the problem succinctly. 4) If it is useful, explain the cause of the system message. 5) Tell the user what to do. 6) Using simple, common words. 7) Use simple illustrations only when they will help (10).

3) **Messages and instructional material be designed and tested for specific patient, caregiver and consumer use cases and contexts.** It is imperative that messages and instructional material be designed and tested for specific patient, caregiver and consumer use cases and contexts in addition to provider use cases and user contexts. As has been discussed above, it is faulty to believe that providers will be using EHRs without using these systems to interact with patients in the context of a clinical encounter or in another way. It should be considered essential to design and test all instructional messages and materials with a reasonable set of representative users to ensure the widest possible safe, appropriate and effective use of EHRs.

4.2.4 Include User Requirements in Product Specifications as a Prerequisite for EHR Certification

To help ensure that the best match is achieved between EHR features and user needs, it is recommended that user requirements be included in all EHR product specifications. This will allow potential users to make informed choices regarding the applicability of a given EHR product for a given set of user needs.

4.3   EHR Evaluation and Monitoring Guidelines

4.3.1 Include Evaluation of EHR Impact on a Target Set of Healthcare Disparities Indicators as a Part of the EHR Effectiveness, Post Adoption and Health Impact Evaluation

All efforts to document the effectiveness of EHR systems should include specific investigation of the EHR impact on healthcare disparities. To facilitate such evaluations, NIST should work in collaboration with the Agency for Healthcare Research and Quality, which currently produces the annual National Healthcare Disparities Report, and other appropriate federal, academic and industry collaborators, to define an EHR healthcare disparities indicator set. Once defined, it should be used as the basis for conducting ongoing Healthcare Disparities Impact Assessments. This work should be supplemented by additional qualitative research among safety net providers and patients from disparity populations to provide additional information regarding the nature, character, quality, magnitude and emergence of new determinants or elimination of current determinants of healthcare disparities impacted by EHR adoption and use.

4.3.2 Implement a National EHR Product Registry

Given the number and diversity of EHR developers and vendors as well as the diverse and dynamic needs of potential EHR users, it is recommended that a National EHR Product Registry be developed for all certified EHR products and other products which in the future are integrated into or otherwise linked with an EHR system. This registry should have standardized reporting requirements as outlined below. This registry would provide significant scientific research, consumer research, product safety and patient educational benefit, for potential EHR customers, users and providers.

EHR Product Reporting Recommendations Targeting EHR Vendors

4.3.2.1 Standardized Technical Elements & Design Feature Reporting

Certified EHR vendors should be required to report a standard set of technical and design features. The reporting requirements should be developed through a consensus driven process of public and private partners including healthcare disparities, disabilities, and underserved population's expertise. Reported data should be publicly available.

4.3.2.2 Product Safety Information Reporting Requirements

Certified EHR vendors should be required to report a standard set of product safety information. Because legacy systems will inevitably be used, this information should remain publicly available even after a particular product is no longer available.

4.3.2.3 Product Evaluation Information Reporting Requirements

Certified EHR vendors should be required to report a standard set of EHR evaluation information. In the future this should include any target user oriented voluntary certifications received by the EHR product. Evaluation information should include information about user requirements and product specifications.

EHR Product Reporting Recommendations Targeting Providers and Healthcare Systems

4.3.2.4 Adverse Event Reporting

The National EHR Registry should facilitate voluntary provider and healthcare system adverse event reporting.

4.3.2.5 Provider Feedback

The National EHR Registry should also facilitate provider feedback regarding the EHR challenges problems, malfunctions, errors experienced while using the system.

EHR Product Reporting Recommendations Targeting Patients, Consumers and Caregiver

4.3.2.6 Patient Education

The National EHR Registry should provide culturally and linguistically appropriate patient educational information regarding certified EHR and associated technology. The information should be supplied by the product vendors but should comply with recognized federal standards for providing Culturally Linguistically Appropriate Services (See Glossary) and communicating information to diverse populations (11).

4.3.2.7 Consumer Feedback

The National EHR Registry should facilitate patient and consumer feedback about EHR systems.

4.4   EHR Research Guidelines

4.4.1   Support Human Factors Research Regarding the Potential Impact, Opportunities and Barriers for EHRs to Reduce Healthcare Disparities

While a significant volume of research has been done regarding user needs and accommodations, particularly in the human factors, ergonomics and disability fields, little of this work has been done from the perspective of healthcare disparities and therefore essentially no human factors and EHR work is found in the healthcare disparities literature. As such, ONC should continue to support research regarding the potential impact, opportunities and barriers for EHRs to reduce Healthcare Disparities as outlined below. These suggestions should not be viewed as an exhaustive nor comprehensive list of research needed to completely understand the human factors impact on healthcare disparities. Rather they represent suggested starting points for future work along these lines.

4.4.2   Evaluate the Human Factors Implications of Integrating Patient-Oriented Functionality into EHRs

Although, as discussed above, several significant policy precedents and initiatives are leading toward the increased patient and consumer use of EHRs, no research has been done to understand the health, healthcare or healthcare disparities implications of enabling consumer engagement with EHRs. Similarly, little is known about the potential value, efficacy or effectiveness of integrating personal health records and other consumer health informatics tools into more traditional EHRs. The evidence base for or against moving in this direction needs to be supported and developed.

4.4.3 Support the Development of Evidence-Based Criteria for Voluntary Population-Oriented Product Certifications

In addition to the recommendations contained in this report and the current evaluation process, it may be valuable to develop and incorporate voluntary user population based EHR evaluation (visually impaired, safety net, etc.). However the evidence base for or against this as a potential mechanism to help address healthcare disparities is currently not available and should be supported.

4.4.4 Evaluate Potential Differences in Information Design Needs, the Impact of These Differences and Opportunities for Accommodation across User Populations

It is not clear whether or not different populations of users (beyond providers and patients) have differing information design needs and whether or not such needs can impact healthcare disparities. Because information architecture is at the heart of any EHR usability, research in this area may have significant importance for addressing healthcare disparities via EHR systems.

4.4.5 Evaluate the Human Factors Implications of Increased Stress (Workload Induced, User Environment Induced, Rural/Urban Residence etc) on EHR Accessibility, Usability, User Experience and Health Outcomes

To date, most of the research regarding stress and human-computer interaction has been done in the context of the work environment. However, as healthcare is increasingly being delivered in the home and community-based setting and as patients increasingly become engaged in their EHRs more research needs to be done to understand the potential impact of the home environment on EHR accessibility, usability, user experience and health outcomes.

4.4.6 Evaluate the Human Factors Implications of the Emerging EHR Health IT Workforce Working in Non Clinical Practice Settings (Home, Long Term Care Facility etc) on EHR Accessibility, Usability, User Experience and Health Outcomes.

A myriad of support personnel will inevitably be EHR system users. These include clinical office/practice managers, receptionist/schedulers and technical support personnel. Without these individuals involved, many providers would not be able to accomplish needed EHR data entry or report/summary requirements and needs. Also there is an emerging health workforce comprised of those individuals who provide or support care primarily in the home and community setting. It is likely that in order to maintain appropriate oversight and management as well as quality assurance and efficiency, these individuals will increasingly be using wireless handheld and tablet or laptop based mobile devices to input data into the HRH in real time, in the field, at the "point of care". The implications of this emerging workforce on Health, healthcare outcomes and healthcare disparities needs to be evaluated.

5 Conclusions

In conclusion, significant scientific evidence attests to the fact that healthcare disparities exist, they are intractable and associated with increased healthcare costs, premature morbidity and excess mortality. Wide adoption and meaningful use of EHRs by providers and patients may impact healthcare disparities. The impact of EHRs on healthcare disparities are almost certainly going to be multifaceted, nuanced, in some cases indirect yet cumulatively significant. These disparities could improve, if EHR use and benefits, are equitably distributed across user populations. On the other hand, disparities could worsen, if some providers are not able to use EHRs or some patients not able to benefit from them.

The fields of human factors engineering and ergonomics have made considerable contributions to our understanding of the possible barriers and potential solutions needed to ensure broad accessibility and usability of emerging EHR systems. Unfortunately, most of this knowledge and expertise, does not appear to be routinely considered during the EHR design and development process (7). In addition, little research along these lines, can be found, in the disparities literature. Few studies of EHR usability or health impact have been done from a healthcare disparities perspective. As such, much more research is warranted. There is also considerable need for federal policy leadership in this area. This leadership will help ensure that all providers are able to use EHRs and also help ensure that all patients are able to benefit from EHR use. Finally, given what is already known, much can be done now to reduce the risk of creating or exacerbating healthcare disparities. Product enhancements can be made by addressing key disparities-related design issues and by incorporating human factors engineering principles into the EHR design and development process. Significant progress along these lines will inevitably improve provider EHR adoption, help lead to reductions in healthcare disparities among affected populations and catalyze improvements in healthcare quality for all.

Glossary

Healthcare Consumers

For the purposes of this report healthcare consumers are defined as individuals do not have a clinical diagnosis provided by a licensed medical professional but who are seeking health information or health related services for the purpose of health maintenance, prevention or wellness

Patients

For the purposes of this report patients are defined as individuals who have an existing clinical diagnosis

Providers

For the purposes of this report providers are defined as any healthcare professional involved in the provision of medical services

Culture

Culture has been variably defined but in terms of the federal CLAS standards it is defined as the thoughts, communications, actions, customs, beliefs, values, and institutions of racial, ethnic, religious, or social groups. Culture defines how health care information is received, how rights and protections are exercised, what is considered to be a health problem, how symptoms and concerns about the problem are expressed, who should provide treatment for the problem, and what type of treatment should be given. (11).

Culturally and Linguistically Appropriate Services (CLAS)

The collective set of CLAS mandates, guidelines, and recommendations issued by the HHS Office of Minority Health intended to inform, guide, and facilitate required and recommended practices related to culturally and linguistically appropriate health services (11).

Culturally and Linguistically Appropriate Services in Health Care

The CLAS standards are proposed as one means to correct inequities that currently exist in the provision of health services and to make these services more responsive to the individual needs of all patients/consumers. The standards are intended to be inclusive of all cultures and not limited to any particular population group or sets of groups. However, they are especially designed to address the needs of racial, ethnic, and linguistic population groups that are medically underserved. Ultimately, the aim of the standards is to contribute to the elimination of racial and ethnic health disparities and to improve the health of all Americans (11).

The CLAS standards serve several purposes. They provide a common understanding and consistent definitions of culturally and linguistically appropriate services in health care. They offer a practical framework for the implementation of services and organizational structures that can help health care organizations and providers be responsive to the cultural and linguistic issues presented by diverse populations (11).

Cultural and linguistic competence is defined as a set of congruent behaviors, attitudes, and policies that come together in a system, agency, or among professionals that enables effective work in cross-cultural situations. 'Competence' implies having the capacity to function effectively as an individual and an organization within the context of the cultural beliefs, behaviors, and needs presented by patients and consumers that are dissimilar to those of one's self." (11)

The CLAS standards are primarily directed at health care organizations; however, individual providers are also encouraged to use the standards to make their practices more culturally and linguistically accessible.

Standard 1. Health care organizations should ensure that patients/consumers receive from all staff members effective, understandable, and respectful care that is provided in a manner compatible with their cultural health beliefs and practices and preferred language.

Standard 2. Health care organizations should implement strategies to recruit, retain, and promote at all levels of the organization a diverse staff and leadership that are representative of the demographic characteristics of the service area.

Standard 3. Health care organizations should ensure that staff at all levels and across all disciplines receive ongoing education and training in culturally and linguistically appropriate service delivery.

Standard 4. Health care organizations must offer and provide language assistance services, including bilingual staff and interpreter services, at no cost to each patient/consumer with limited English proficiency at all points of contact, in a timely manner during all hours of operation.

Standard 5. Health care organizations must provide to patients/consumers in their preferred language both verbal offers and written notices informing them of their right to receive language assistance services.

Standard 6. Health care organizations must assure the competence of language assistance provided to limited English proficient patients/consumers by interpreters and bilingual staff. Family and friends should not be used to provide interpretation services (except on request by the patient/consumer).

Standard 7. Health care organizations must make available easily understood patient-related materials and post signage in the languages of the commonly encountered groups and/or groups represented in the service area.

Standard 8. Health care organizations should develop, implement, and promote a written strategic plan that outlines clear goals, policies, operational plans, and management accountability/oversight mechanisms to provide culturally and linguistically appropriate services.

Standard 9. Health care organizations should conduct initial and ongoing organizational self-assessments of CLAS-related activities and are encouraged to integrate cultural and linguistic competence-related measures into their internal audits, performance improvement programs, patient satisfaction assessments, and outcomes-based evaluations.

Standard 10. Health care organizations should ensure that data on the individual patients/consumer's race, ethnicity, and spoken and written language are collected in health records, integrated into the organization's management information systems, and periodically updated.

Standard 11. Health care organizations should maintain a current demographic, cultural, and epidemiological profile of the community as well as a needs assessment to accurately plan for and implement services that respond to the cultural and linguistic characteristics of the service area.

Standard 12. Health care organizations should develop participatory, collaborative partnerships with communities and utilize a variety of formal and informal mechanisms to facilitate community and patient/consumer involvement in designing and implementing CLAS-related activities.

Standard 13. Health care organizations should ensure that conflict and grievance resolution processes are culturally and linguistically sensitive and capable of identifying, preventing, and resolving cross-cultural conflicts or complaints by patients/consumers.

Standard 14. Health care organizations are encouraged to regularly make available to the public information about their progress and successful innovations in implementing the CLAS standards and to provide public notice in their communities about the availability of this information.

Healthcare Disparities

The Institute of Medicine defines healthcare disparities as differences in the quality of healthcare received by patients that is not due to access-related factors, clinical need, preferences or appropriateness of the health intervention (14). The causes of these disparities have not been definitively characterized. General consensus holds them to be related to population differences in 1) environmental exposures, 2) healthcare access, utilization and/or quality of care, (3). Within the U.S. healthcare system, these differences have most convincingly been demonstrated across racial and ethnic lines (Whites vs. minorities) (14). However other categorizations including geographic (urban vs. rural) (106), gender (male vs. female) (107;108), disability (disabled vs. non-disabled) (109-111), socioeconomic status (poor vs. non-poor) (55;112), and age (non-elderly vs. elderly) (113;114) have also been described (3). Some authorities have sought to cast a distinction between healthcare disparities defined above and health disparities which have been defined population differences in health status that are thought to be related to broader societal factors (education, poverty, employment, stress etc) (115;116). The Institute of Medicine definition will be used for the purposes of this report (14).

Safety Net Providers

Safety net providers have been defined as those who deliver a significant level of health care to uninsured, Medicaid, and other vulnerable patients (6). In addition, core safety net providers have two distinguishing characteristics. They (1) by legal mandate or explicitly adopted mission they maintain an "open door," offering access to services to patients regardless of their ability to pay; and (2) a substantial share of their patient mix is uninsured, Medicaid, and other vulnerable patients. Core providers include a variety of health centers (e.g., community health centers, migrant health centers, the Health Care for the Homeless Program, school-based health centers, community-based clinics, public hospitals, and many teaching hospitals) (6). A substantial amount of safety net care is provided in hospital emergency departments, which, as a condition of participation in the federal Medicare program, are required to provide medical screening exams and stabilizing treatment to all patients, regardless of their ability to pay. In addition, a considerable, but largely unquantified, amount of health care for safety net populations is provided in private physicians' offices.

Usability

Usability is the effectiveness, efficiency, and satisfaction with which specific patients and providers can achieve a specific set of tasks in a particular environment. Ease of learning is also a component of usability. Efficiency is generally the speed with which patients and providers can complete their tasks. Effectiveness is the accuracy and completeness with which patients and providers can complete tasks. This includes how easy it is for patients and providers to make errors. User errors can lead to inaccurate or incomplete patient records, can alter provider clinical decision-making, patient self management decision-making and can compromise patient safety. User satisfaction is usually the first concept people think of in relation to "usability." Satisfaction in the context of usability refers to the subjective satisfaction a user may have with a process or outcome. Efficiency, effectiveness, and satisfaction cannot be taken in isolation— all three components must be evaluated and balanced based on your practice's goals and priorities (117).

Usability in the context of this report has little to do with the visual appeal of the user EHR system interface. Applications that use lots of colors or visual elements probably would have a lower usability "score" than well thought out designs that are simpler in appearance. Thoughtful use of visual elements can be a supporting factor that helps enhance product usability. Additional usability factors that must be considered in the design and development of EHRs, to prevent disparities among diverse patients and providers includes "ease of use" and "user experience." EHR systems are complex systems dealing with sensitive and sometimes confusing information. In terms of ensuring usability of these systems there is great need to analyze, test and address difficult aspects of EHR use such as counter intuitive interactions, confusing, misleading, or overly complex EHR system interface characteristics, logic of operation, differences from user expectations, - any of which could possibly lead to harm to patients or impact patient outcomes (118).

The term "accessibility" refers to design criteria, which remove barriers that make it difficult or impossible for some people with disabilities to use HIT. The intent behind accessibility is to implement the principle of non-discrimination. It is a way of demonstrating that healthcare entities (such as organizations, providers, academic institutions and companies) wish to be welcoming to all people, including people with disabilities (118).

User-Centered Design

User-centered design (UCD) is an approach to interactive system development that focuses specifically on making systems usable. It is a multi-disciplinary activity which incorporates human factors and ergonomics knowledge and techniques. The application of human factors and ergonomics to interactive systems design, enhances effectiveness and efficiency, improves human working conditions, and counteracts possible adverse effects of use on human health, safety and performance. Applying ergonomics to the design of systems involves taking account of human capabilities, skills, limitations and needs (117).

A plan should be developed to specify how the human-centered activities fit into the overall system development process. The plan should identify: a) the context of EHR use, specifying user and organizational requirements, producing prototypes and evaluating designs according to user criteria; b) procedures for integrating these activities with other system development activities, e.g. analysis, design, testing; c) the individuals and the organization(s) responsible for the human-centered design activities and the range of skills and viewpoints they provide; d) effective procedures for establishing feedback and communication on human-centered design activities as they affect other design activities, and methods for documenting these activities; e) appropriate milestones for human-centered activities integrated into the overall design and development process; f) suitable timescales to allow feedback, and possible design changes, to be incorporated into the project schedule (117).

Making systems more usable means systems can contribute to organizational aims and meet user and organizational needs better. Using a UCD approach can result in EHR systems that are easier to understand and use, thus reducing training and support costs. It can also improve user satisfaction and reduce discomfort and stress as well as improve the productivity and operational efficiency of organizations. Finally, it can also improve product quality, appeal to the patients and providers and can provide a competitive advantage. The complete benefits of human-centered design can be determined by taking into account the total life-cycle costs of the system including conception, design, implementation, support, use and maintenance (117).

Feedback from patients and providers is a critical source of information in user-centered design. Evaluating designs with patients and providers and improving them based on their feedback provides an effective means of minimizing the risk of a system not meeting user or organizational needs (including those requirements that are hidden or difficult to specify explicitly). Such evaluation allows preliminary design solutions to be tested against "real world" scenarios, with the results being fed back into progressively refined solutions. It is important to keep in mind that these evaluations need to be performed from the provider and patients perspectives.

The most appropriate design cannot typically be achieved without iteration or without repeating a sequence of steps, until a desired outcome is achieved. This may be done at multiple points in the developmental cycle. User-centered activities can be iterated for individual parts of the EHR development process and again at a completed whole system level. Iteration should be used to progressively eliminate uncertainty during the development of interactive systems. Iteration implies that descriptions, specifications and prototypes are revised and refined when new information is obtained in order to minimize the risk of the system under development failing to meet user requirements (17).

The complexity of provider-EHR-patient interactions means that it is impossible to specify completely and accurately every detail, of every aspect, of the interaction, at the beginning of development. Many of the needs and expectations of provider, patients and caregivers that will impact on the design of the interaction, only emerge in the course of development, as the designers refine their understanding of the patients and providers and their tasks, or as patients and providers are better able to express their needs in response to potential solutions. Iteration of proposed solutions incorporating feedback from a user perspective provides a means of mitigating risk (17).

Using a user-centered approach to EHR design and development has substantial economic and social benefits for patients and providers, employers and suppliers. Highly usable systems and products tend to be more successful both technically and commercially (17). Support and help-desk costs are reduced when patients and providers can understand and use products without additional assistance. In most countries, employers and suppliers have legal obligations to protect patients and providers from risks to their health, and safety and user-centered methods can reduce these risks.

Universal Accessibility

The term "accessibility" in the context of this report refers to design criteria, which remove barriers that make it difficult or impossible for some people with disabilities to use HIT. Universal

Accessibility focuses on removing barriers to utilization such that anyone can have the ability to use health IT. From this perspective, accessibility can be viewed as a means toward reducing healthcare disparities or achieving health equity in health IT or EHR access. Accessible HIT supports the needs of people with a variety of needs (118).

Universal Usability

Universal Usability is a design philosophy that attempts to make technology usable by all by focusing on a) user diversity, b) technology diversity c) bridging the gap between what users know and what they need to know (119). User diversity focuses on the variety of potential users, including those with different skills, knowledge, age, gender, disabilities, disabling conditions (mobility, sunlight, noise), literacy, culture, income, and so forth (9). Technology diversity focuses on using the most appropriate technologies (i.e. desktop computers, laptop computers, kiosks, tablets, mobile devices using various screen sizes and internet connection speeds) Conceptually, Universal Usability means designing for the purpose of enabling every user to successfully use a given technology. Universal usability is often confused with universal access, which merely means having the equipment/technology and opportunity to use (119). There are many ways to fill the gap between what patients know and what they need to know about using health IT. Technology examples would include help menus or frequently asked questions. Accommodating a broader spectrum of usage situations require designers to consider a wider range of designs, but it also often leads to innovations that benefit all users (9).

While critics of Universal Usability exist, a recent Rand Corporation report on universal access made it clear that "better understanding of the capabilities and limitations of current user-computer interfaces is needed." In addition a National Academy of Science/National Research Council panel on every-citizen interfaces has recommended that "an aggressive universal usability research program, funded by government and private sources, that examines both the human performance side of interfaces and the interface technologies, current and future potential" be established (9). This report and subsequent federal efforts to research, evaluate and ensure Universal access and usability in the area of EHR systems represents a critical component of the Federal Governments' leadership along these lines.

Disclaimer

Any mention of commercial products or reference to commercial organizations is for information only; it does not imply recommendation or endorsement by NIST nor does it imply that the products mentioned are necessarily the best available for the purpose.

Reference List

(1) Committee on Quality of Health Care in America. Crossing the Quality Chasm. Washington DC: National Academy Press, 2001.

(2) Calman N, Kitson K, Hauser D. Using Information Technology to Improve Health Quality and Safety in Community Health Centers. Prog Community Health Partnersh 2007; 1(1):83-88.

(3) Gibbons MC. A historical overview of health disparities and the potential of eHealth solutions. J Med Internet Res 2005; 7(5):e50.

(4) Ketcham JD, Lutfey KE, Gerstenberger E, Link CL, McKinlay JB. Physician clinical information technology and health care disparities. Med Care Res Rev 2009; 66(6):658-681.

(5) EHR adoption rate in U.S. physician offices increases 3.2% since 2009. http://www.healthimaging.com/index.php?option=com_articles&view=article&id=206 93:ehr-adoption-rate-in-us-physician-offices-increases-32-since-2009 . 2010.
Ref Type: Electronic Citation

(6) Gibbons MC, Casale C.R. Reducing disparities in healthcare quality: The role of Health IT in underresourced settings. Med Care Res Rev 2010; 67:155S-165S.

(7) McDonnell C, Werner K, Wendel L. Electronic Health Record Usability Vendor Practices and Perspectives. 09(10)-0091-3-EF. 2010. Rockville, MD, The Agency for Healthcare Research and Quality.
Ref Type: Report

(8) Joint Technical Committee ISO/IEC JTC 1. Software engineering — Software product Quality Requirements and Evaluation (SQuaRE) — Common Industry Format (CIF) for usability test reports. ISO/IEC 25062. 2006. Switzerland, The International Organization for Standardization and The International Electrotechnical Commission.
Ref Type: Report

(9) Shneiderman B. Universal Usability. Communications of the ACM 2000; 43(5).

(10) Redish J, Laskowski S. Guidelines for Writing Clear Instructions and Messages for Voters and Poll Workers. NISTIR 7596. 2009. Gaithersburg, MD, National Institute of Standards and Technology.
Ref Type: Report

(11) National Standards for Culturally and LinguisticallyAppropriate Services in Health Care. 2001. Washington, DC, DHHS, OPHS, Office of Minority Health.
Ref Type: Report

(12) Rosenthal TC. The medical home: growing evidence to support a new approach to primary care. J Am Board Fam Med 2008; 21(5):427-440.

(13) President's vision for Health IT. http://www.hhs.gov/healthit/presvision.html . 2005.
Ref Type: Electronic Citation

(14) Committee on understanding and eliminating racial and ethnic disparities in health care. Unequal Treatment; Confronting Racial and Ethnic Disparities in Health Care. 2002. Washington DC, National Academies Press.
Ref Type: Report

(15) Waidmann T. Estimating the Cost of Racial and Ethnic Health Disparities. 2009. Washington, DC, The Urban Institute.
Ref Type: Report

(16) LaVeist T, Gaskin D, Richard P. The Economic burden of Health inequalities in the United States. 2009. Washington, DC, The Joint Center for Political and Economic Studies.
Ref Type: Report

(17) Ergonomics of human–system interaction — Part 210: Human-centred design for interactive systems. ISO 9241-210. 2010. Switzerland, International Standards Organization.
Ref Type: Report

(18) McPherson K, Wennberg JE, Hovind OB, Clifford P. Small-area variations in the use of common surgical procedures: an international comparison of New England, England, and Norway. N Engl J Med 1982; 307(21):1310-1314.

(19) Barnes BA, O'Brien E, Comstock C, D'Arpa DG, Donahue CL. Report on variation in rates of utilization of surgical services in the Commonwealth of Massachusetts. JAMA 1985; 254(3):371-375.

(20) Department of Health and Human Services. Report of the Secretary's Task Forces on Black and Minority Health. 1985. Washington, DC, DHHS.
Ref Type: Report

(21) Marmot MG. Does stress cause heart attacks? Postgrad Med J 1986; 62(729):683-686.

(22) Sapolsky RM, Mott GE. Social subordinance in wild baboons is associated with suppressed high density lipoprotein-cholesterol concentrations: the possible role of chronic social stress. Endocrinology 1987; 121(5):1605-1610.

(23) Tager IB, Weiss ST, Munoz A, Rosner B, Speizer FE. Longitudinal study of the effects of maternal smoking on pulmonary function in children. N Engl J Med 1983; 309(12):699-703.

(24) Kawachi I, Kennedy BP, Lochner K, Prothrow-Stith D. Social capital, income inequality, and mortality. Am J Public Health 1997; 87(9):1491-1498.

(25) Wilkinson RG. Comment: income, inequality, and social cohesion. Am J Public Health 1997; 87(9):1504-1506.

(26) Shi L, Starfield B, Kennedy B, Kawachi I. Income inequality, primary care, and health indicators. J Fam Pract 1999; 48(4):275-284.

(27) Wilkinson RG. Income inequality and population health. Soc Sci Med 1998; 47(3):411-412.

(28) Coverdell M, Utley R. Health Care Information Gap: A Global and National Perspective. Online Journal of Nursing Informatics 2005; 9(1).

(29) The Agency for Healthcare Research and Quality. The National Healthcare Disparities Report 2009. 2010. Washington DC, AHRQ.
Ref Type: Report

(30) Shrestha L. The Changing Demographic Profile of the United States. RL32701. 2006. Washington, DC, *Congressional Research Service - The Library of Congress*.
Ref Type: Report

(31) Trends in aging--United States and worldwide. MMWR Morb Mortal Wkly Rep 2003; 52(6):101-4, 106.

(32) Hing E, Burt CW. Are there patient disparities when electronic health records are adopted? J Health Care Poor Underserved 2009; 20(2):473-488.

(33) Ramaiah M, Subrahmanian E, Sriram R, Lide B. Workflow and Electronic Health Records in Small Medical Practices. NISTIR 7732. 2010. Alexandria, VA, US Department of Comerce.
Ref Type: Report

(34) Gibbons MC, Wilson RF, Samal L, Lehman CU, Dickersin K, Lehmann HP et al. Impact of consumer health informatics applications. (Prepared by Johns Hopkins Evidence Based Practice Center Under contract No.HHSA 290-2007-10061-I), editor. Evid.Rep.Technol.Assess.(Full.Rep.) 09(10)-E019[188], 1-546. 2009.
Ref Type: Report

(35) Carpenter WR, Godley PA, Clark JA, Talcott JA, Finnegan T, Mishel M et al. Racial differences in trust and regular source of patient care and the implications for prostate cancer screening use. Cancer 2009; 115(21):5048-5059.

(36) Shi L, Stevens GD. Vulnerability and unmet health care needs. The influence of multiple risk factors. J Gen Intern Med 2005; 20(2):148-154.

(37) Alegria M, Sribney W, Perez D, Laderman M, Keefe K. The role of patient activation on patient-provider communication and quality of care for US and foreign born Latino patients. J Gen Intern Med 2009; 24 Suppl 3:534-541.

(38) Ratanawongsa N, Zikmund-Fisher BJ, Couper MP, Van Hoewyk J, Powe NR. Race, ethnicity, and shared decision making for hyperlipidemia and hypertension treatment: the DECISIONS survey. Med Decis Making 2010; 30(5 Suppl):65S-76S.

(39) Peek ME, Odoms-Young A, Quinn MT, Gorawara-Bhat R, Wilson SC, Chin MH. Race and shared decision-making: perspectives of African-Americans with diabetes. Soc Sci Med 2010; 71(1):1-9.

(40) Peek ME, Wilson SC, Gorawara-Bhat R, Odoms-Young A, Quinn MT, Chin MH. Barriers and facilitators to shared decision-making among African-Americans with diabetes. J Gen Intern Med 2009; 24(10):1135-1139.

(41) Epstein RM, Fiscella K, Lesser CS, Stange KC. Why the nation needs a policy push on patient-centered health care. Health Aff (Millwood) 2010; 29(8):1489-1495.

(42) Institute of Medicine (US) Forum on the Science of Health Care Quality Improvement and Implementation, Institute of Medicine (US) Roundtable on Health Disparities, Institute of Medicine (US) Roundtable on Health Literacy. Toward Health Equity and Patient-Centeredness: Integrating Health Literacy, Disparities Reduction, and Quality Improvement: Workshop Summary. 2009. Washington, DC, National Academies Press.
Ref Type: Report

(43) Mandl KD, Kohane IS, Brandt AM. Electronic patient-physician communication: problems and promise. Ann Intern Med 1998; 129(6):495-500.

(44) Roblin DW, Houston TK, Allison JJ, Joski PJ, Becker ER. Disparities in use of a personal health record in a managed care organization. J Am Med Inform Assoc 2009; 16(5):683-689.

(45) Pagliari C, Detmer D, Singleton P. Potential of electronic personal health records. BMJ 2007; 335(7615):330-333.

(46) Wolf MS, Wilson EA, Rapp DN, Waite KR, Bocchini MV, Davis TC et al. Literacy and learning in health care. Pediatrics 2009; 124 Suppl 3:S275-S281.

(47) Rothman RL, Yin HS, Mulvaney S, Co JP, Homer C, Lannon C. Health literacy and quality: focus on chronic illness care and patient safety. Pediatrics 2009; 124 Suppl 3:S315-S326.

(48) LaVeist TA, Isaac LA, Williams KP. Mistrust of Health Care Organizations Is Associated with Underutilization of Health Services. Health Serv Res 2009.

(49) Nguyen GC, LaVeist TA, Harris ML, Datta LW, Bayless TM, Brant SR. Patient trust-in-physician and race are predictors of adherence to medical management in inflammatory bowel disease. Inflamm Bowel Dis 2009; 15(8):1233-1239.

(50) Arora NK, Gustafson DH. Perceived helpfulness of physicians' communication behavior and breast cancer patients' level of trust over time. J Gen Intern Med 2009; 24(2):252-255.

(51) Kennedy BR, Mathis CC, Woods AK. African Americans and their distrust of the health care system: healthcare for diverse populations. J Cult Divers 2007; 14(2):56-60.

(52) Boulware LE, Cooper LA, Ratner LE, LaVeist TA, Powe NR. Race and trust in the health care system. Public Health Rep 2003; 118(4):358-365.

(53) Manhattan Research. Cybercitizen Health v9.0. 2010. New York, NY, Manhattan Research.
Ref Type: Report

(54) Korzenny F, Vann L. Tapping into their connections: The multicultural world of social media marketing. 2009. Tallahassee, FL, Florida State University Center for Hispanic Marketing Communication.
Ref Type: Report

(55) DeNavas-Walt C, Proctor B, Smith J. Income, Poverty, and Health Insurance Coverage in the United States: 2009. Current Population Reports, P60-238. 2010. Washington, DC, US Census Bereau.
Ref Type: Report

(56) Hing E, Hsiao CJ. Electronic medical record use by office-based physicians and their practices: United States, 2007. Natl Health Stat Report 2010;(23):1-11.

(57) Baker DW. Reading between the lines: deciphering the connections between literacy and health. J Gen Intern Med 1999; 14(5):315-317.

(58) About the CAHPS Item Set for Addressing Health Literacy. https://www.cahps.ahrq.gov/CAHPSkit/files/1311_About_Health_Lit.pdf Document No.1311 . 2009.
Ref Type: Electronic Citation

(59) Williams MV, Parker RM, Baker DW, Parikh NS, Pitkin K, Coates WC et al. Inadequate functional health literacy among patients at two public hospitals. JAMA: The Journal of the American Medical Association 1995; 274(21):1677-1682.

(60) Baker DW. Reading between the lines: deciphering the connections between literacy and health. J Gen Intern Med 1999; 14(5):315-317.

(61) Baquis D. Health Information Technology Accessability for Persons with Disabilities. In: Kahn S, Hickner J, editors. A Community view:How personal health records can improve patient care and outcomes in many healthcare settings. Northern Illinois University Regional Development Institute, 2008: 146-152.

(62) Disability Evaluation Under Social Security (Blue Book- September 2008).
  http://www.ssa.gov/disability/professionals/bluebook/general-info.htm . 2008.
Ref Type: Electronic Citation

(63) Disabilities. http://www.who.int/topics/disabilities/en/ . 2010. The World
  HealthOrganization.
Ref Type: Electronic Citation

(64) Kochkin S. MarkeTrak VIII: 25-Year Trends in the Hearing Health Market. The Hearing
  Review 2009; 16(11):12-31.

(65) Encyclopedia of Disability. Thousand Oaks, CA: Sage Publishers, 2005.

(66) Disabled World. Physical and Mobility Impairments. http://www.disabled-
  world.com/disability/types/mobility/#ixzz13IAuHfz2 . 2010.
Ref Type: Electronic Citation

(67) Web Accessibility for Older Users: A Literature Review. Arch A, editor. 2008. World
  Wide Web Consortium.
Ref Type: Report

(68) TITLE XVI-Supplemental Security Income for the Aged, Blind and Disabled.
  http://www.ssa.gov/OP_Home/ssact/title16b/1614.htm . 2010. Social Security
  Administration.
Ref Type: Electronic Citation

(69) American FOundation for the Blind. Low Vision.
  http://www.afb.org/Section.asp?SectionID=93 . 2010.
Ref Type: Electronic Citation

(70) Disabilities Sourcebook. Omnigraphics, 2001.

(71) Stone M, Laskowski S, Lowery S. Guidelines for Using Color in Voting Systems. NISTIR
  7537 . 2008. Gaithersburg, MD, National institute of Standards and Technology.
Ref Type: Report

(72) Disabled World. Cognitive Disabilities. http://www.disabled-
  world.com/disability/types/cognitive/ . 2010.
Ref Type: Electronic Citation

(73) Cognitive Disabilities. http://webaim.org/articles/cognitive/ . 2010. Center for Persons
  with DIsabilities at Utah State University.
Ref Type: Electronic Citation

(74) Meyer J. Age 2000. 2001. Washington, DC, US Census Bureau.
Ref Type: Report

(75) Hedden T, Gabrieli JD. Insights into the ageing mind: a view from cognitive neuroscience. Nat Rev Neurosci 2004; 5(2):87-96.

(76) Nilsson LG. Memory function in normal aging. Acta Neurol Scand Suppl 2003; 179:7-13.

(77) Johnson MK, Reeder JA, Raye CL, Mitchell KJ. Second thoughts versus second looks: an age-related deficit in reflectively refreshing just-activated information. Psychol Sci 2002; 13(1):64-67.

(78) Johnson MK, Hashtroudi S, Lindsay DS. Source monitoring. Psychol Bull 1993; 114(1):3-28.

(79) Mitchell KJ, Johnson MK, Raye CL, Mather M, D'Esposito M. Aging and reflective processes of working memory: binding and test load deficits. Psychol Aging 2000; 15(3):527-541.

(80) Caserta R, Abrams L. The relevance of situation awareness in older adults' cognitive functioning: a review. Aging and Physical Activity 2007; 4:3-13.

(81) Holden T, Adolf J. Human-Computer Interface (HCI) Design Guide. 1995. Houston, TX, National Aeronautics and Space Administration.
Ref Type: Report

(82) O'Hara J, Brown W, Lewis P, Persensky J. Human-System Interface Design Review Guidelines. NUREG-0700. 2002. Washington, DC, U.S. Nuclear Regulatory Commission.
Ref Type: Report

(83) Wickens C. Multiple Resources and Mental Workload. Human Factors: The Journal of the Human Factors and Ergonomics Society 2008; 50:449.

(84) Jimison H, Gorman P, Woods S, Nygren P, Walker M, Norris S et al. Barriers and drivers of health information technology use for the elderly, chronically ill, and underserved. Evid Rep Technol Assess (Full Rep) 2008;(175):1-1422.

(85) Lober WB, Zierler B, Herbaugh A, Shinstrom SE, Stolyar A, Kim EH et al. Barriers to the use of a personal health record by an elderly population. AMIA Annu Symp Proc 2006;514-518.

(86) Jha AK, Bates DW, Jenter C, Orav EJ, Zheng J, Cleary P et al. Electronic health records: use, barriers and satisfaction among physicians who care for black and Hispanic patients. J Eval Clin Pract 2009; 15(1):158-163.

(87) Murchinson JV, Apodaca A, Sison CE, Rosenberg C, Swafford R. For the record: EHR adoption in the safety net. 1-46. 2-1-2009. The California Healthcare Foundation.
Ref Type: Report

(88) Castenda JA, Mun~oz-Leiva F, Luque T. Web Acceptance Model (WAM): Moderating effects of user experience. Information & Management 2007; 44:384-396.

(89) Gamm L, Hutchinson L, Dabney B, Dorsey A. Rural Healthy People 2010; A Companion document to Health People 2010. 2003. College Station, TX, Texas A& M Health Sciences Center.
Ref Type: Report

(90) National Rural Health Association. http://www.ruralhealthweb.org/go/left/about-rural-health/what-s-different-about-rural-health-care . 2010.
Ref Type: Electronic Citation

(91) Bahensky JA, Jaana M, Ward MM. Health care information technology in rural America: electronic medical record adoption status in meeting the national agenda. J Rural Health 2008; 24(2):101-105.

(92) Mansfeld M. Recognizing ergonomics variations: Human factors in technology transfer to newly industrializing countries. Jounrnal of Technology Transfer 1987; 11(2):19-27.

(93) Smith-Jackson T, Wogalter M. Applying cultural ergonomics/Human Factors to safety information research. Proceedings of the IEA /2OOO/HFES 2000 Congress , 6-150-6-153. 2000. Santa Monica, CA, Human Factors and Ergonomics Society.
Ref Type: Report

(94) Technical Committee ISO/TC 215 HiWG1Hramc. Health informatics — Electronic health record — Definition, scope, and context. ISO/TR 20514:2005(E). 2005. Geneva, Switzerland, International Organization for Standardization (ISO).
Ref Type: Report

(95) Armijo D, McDonnell C, Werner K. Electronic Health Record Usability Evaluation and Use Case Framework. **09(10)-0091-1-EF** . 2009. Rockville, MD, Agency for Healthcare Research and Quality.
Ref Type: Report

(96) Brown C. Human factors problems in the design and evaluation of key-entry devices for the Japanese language. In: Chapanis A, editor. Ethnic Variables in Human Factors Engineering. Baltimore, MD: Johns Hopkins University Press, 1975.

(97) Hsu S, Peng Y. Control display relationship of the 4-burner stove – a reexamination. Human Factors: The Journal of the Human Factors and Ergonomics Society 1993; 35(4):745-749.

(98) Courney A. Chinese population stereotypes – color associations. Human Factors: The Journal of the Human Factors and Ergonomics Society 1986; 28(1):97-99.

(99) Choong Y, Salvendy G. Design of icons for use by Chinese in mainland China. Ineract Comput 1998; 9(4):417-430.

(100) Dong J, Salvendy G. Designing menus for the Chinese population: horizontal or vertical? Behav Inform Technol 1999; 18(6):467-471.

(101) Fang X, Rau P. Culture differences in design of portal sites. Ergonomics 2003; 46(1-3):242-254.

(102) Shen S, Woolley M, Prior S. Towards culture-centered design. Interacting with Computers 2006; 18(4):820-852.

(103) Forsythe D. New Bottles, Old Wine: Hidden Cultural Assumptions in a Computerized Explanation System for Migraine Sufferers. Medical Anthropology Quarterly 1996; 10(4):551-574.

(104) Downey S, Wentling R, Wentling T, Wadsworth A. The Relationship Between National Culture and the Usability of an E-Learning System. 871-878. 2004. Champaign, IL, University of Illinois at Urbana-Champaign.
Ref Type: Report

(105) Lansky D, Kanaan S, Lemieux J. Identifying Appropriate Federal Roles in the Development of Electronic Personal Health Records: Results of a Key Informant Process: Results of a Key Informant Process. http://odphp.osophs.dhhs.gov/projects/PHRecords/default.htm . 2005. DHHS Ofice of Disease Prevention and Health Promotion.
Ref Type: Electronic Citation

(106) Verheij RA. Explaining urban-rural variations in health: a review of interactions between individual and environment. Soc Sci Med 1996; 42(6):923-935.

(107) Wilkosz ME, Chen JL, Kennedy C, Rankin S. Gender and ethnic disparities contributing to overweight in California adolescents. Z Gesundh Wiss 2010; 18(2):131-144.

(108) Paggi MG, Vona R, Abbruzzese C, Malorni W. Gender-related disparities in non-small cell lung cancer. Cancer Lett 2010; 298(1):1-8.

(109) Rosso AL, Wisdom JP, Horner-Johnson W, McGee MG, Michael YL. Aging with a disability: A systematic review of cardiovascular disease and osteoporosis among women aging with a physical disability. Maturitas 2010.

(110) Wisdom JP, McGee MG, Horner-Johnson W, Michael YL, Adams E, Berlin M. Health disparities between women with and without disabilities: a review of the research. Soc Work Public Health 2010; 25(3):368-386.

(111) Iezzoni LI, Ngo LH, Li D, Roetzheim RG, Drews RE, McCarthy EP. Treatment disparities for disabled medicare beneficiaries with stage I non-small cell lung cancer. Arch Phys Med Rehabil 2008; 89(4):595-601.

(112) LaVeist TA, Thorpe RJ, Jr., Galarraga JE, Bower KM, Gary-Webb TL. Environmental and socio-economic factors as contributors to racial disparities in diabetes prevalence. J Gen Intern Med 2009; 24(10):1144-1148.

(113) Gross SM, Gary TL, Browne DC, LaVeist TA. Gender differences in body image and health perceptions among graduating seniors from a historically black college. J Natl Med Assoc 2005; 97(12):1608-1619.

(114) Wiggins CL, Harlan LC, Nelson HE, Stevens JL, Willman CL, Libby EN et al. Age disparity in the dissemination of imatinib for treating chronic myeloid leukemia. Am J Med 2010; 123(8):764-769.

(115) Carter-Pokras O, Baquet C. What is a "health disparity"? Public Health Rep 2002; 117(5):426-434.

(116) Adler NE, Rehkopf DH. U.S. disparities in health: descriptions, causes, and mechanisms. Annu Rev Public Health 2008; 29:235-252.

(117) Shneiderman B. Universal useability: Designing computer interfaces for diverse users. Hoboken NJ: John Wiley & Sons, Ltd., 2007.

(118) Baquis D. Comments on HITECH Initial Set Interim Final Rule. 5-5-2010. Office of the National Coordinator Health IT Policy Committee.
Ref Type: Hearing

(119) Universal usability: Designing computer interfaces for diverse user populations. Hoboken NJ: John Wiley & Sons, Ltd., 2007.